FIGHTING CANCER

When his wife Bernadette was diagnosed with cancer, Jonathan Chamberlain vowed to find out as much as he could about the disease. What he discovered shocked him. He found that doctors are pursuing treatments that are damaging patients in large numbers often with little possibility of curing them. On the other hand, alternative forms of treatment that appear to have exciting results – while being totally harmless – are ignored.

Jonathan Chamberlain read book after book in his own search for a solution to his wife's illness. Each contained interesting information, but none provided the all-encompassing context that allowed a proper comparison of standard medical and complementary or alternative treatments.

This book, begun after his wife's death, contains the answers Jonathan arrived at. In his view, every adult is responsible for making his or her own decisions about what treatments they wish to choose, but this responsibility can only be properly exercised if information is available and accessible. *Fighting Cancer* provides this information, and is a primer in basic cancer literacy.

Since one person in two will get cancer at some time in their lives, Jonathan believes that people should inform themselves about this disease and the range of possible treatments *before* they get cancer.

Jonathan Chamberlain is a teacher, writer and activist for mental handicap charities. He lives in Hong Kong with his son Patrick.

FIGHTING CANCER
A Survival Guide

Jonathan Chamberlain

HEADLINE

First published in 1997
by HEADLINE BOOK PUBLISHING

10 9 8 7 6 5 4 3 2 1

ISBN 0 7472 7728 1

Typeset by
Letterpart Limited, Reigate, Surrey

Printed and bound in Great Britain by
Mackays of Chatham PLC, Chatham, Kent

HEADLINE BOOK PUBLISHING
A division of Hodder Headline PLC
338 Euston Road
London NW1 3BH

This book is dedicated to the memory of Bernadette Sau-fong, for whom it was too late.

Contents

Acknowledgements

This book is dedicated to my wife, Bernadette Sau-fong, and I must also acknowledge a great debt to her extraordinary courage and grace in the face of her continual pain, her ultimate acceptance of imminent death and her fortitude in keeping death at bay while the family arrived from distant corners of the world to be with her. I owe her more than even I know.

I also owe a profound debt to Vicky Parker, who supplied detailed comments on the chapter on radiation, and whose commentary enabled me to avoid many errors. Vicky is one of the founders of RAGE (Radiotherapy Action Group Exposure), an organisation created by radiation-damaged patients who are seeking a wider understanding of their plight. In recognition of the value of her support, RAGE will receive five per cent of my royalties from this book.

In writing this book, I have been very fortunate in having the library resources of the Hong Kong Cancer Fund. Without access to these books, it is unlikely I would have been able to start work on this project.

I wish also to acknowledge the invaluable help of Edith Segall, who commented very usefully on the chapter on homeopathy; of Annette Crisswell, who added information on support groups; of Gary Oden, who talked to me about his wife's successful fight so far against her breast cancer; of David Wilkinson, who supplied background information on the current state of legal rights for patients; and of cancer survivor Hazel Thornton, who corresponded with me. Thanks also to Charles Ha and Alan and Martha Cheng for supplying books and information on supplements from Canada.

Lastly, I must thank my agent, Pam Dix, for the efforts she has put into commenting on, editing and marketing this book; and Susan Fleming, Health Editor, whose commitment to the project has been very encouraging.

The object of *Fighting Cancer* is to provide information on cancer treatments – both orthodox and complementary – not to be a substitute for professional care. Because each person and each situation is unique, the author and publishers urge you to seek appropriate medical advice for your own condition. None of the treatments mentioned in this book is advocated for any individual.

Foreword for people who don't (yet?) have cancer

Why should you read this book? Because it is one hundred per cent certain that you – or someone close to you – will get cancer. The incidence of cancer is rising inexorably, as the following statistics show.

Early 1800s: One in fifty deaths attributed to cancer.

1900: One in twenty-seven.

1920: 'One Out of Every Ten Persons Over Forty Dies of Cancer' – American Society for the Control of Cancer poster (1919). (This was a scare tactic – the actual death toll was one in sixteen.)

1930: One in twelve.

1940: One in nine.

1950: One in seven.

1960: 'According to present government statistics, one out of every six persons in our population will die of cancer. It will not be long before the entire population will have to decide whether we will all die of cancer or change fundamentally all our living and nutritional conditions.' (Max Gerson, author of *A Cancer Therapy*, 1958)

1980: 'If the present trend continues, at least one in four of us will contract cancer. One in five will die of the disease.' (Ralph Moss, author of *The Cancer Industry*, 1982)

1993: 'Cancer may be the most feared disease of our time. It is second only to heart disease as a leading cause of death in the United States, and it is estimated that one in every three Americans will develop cancer at some point in their lives.' (Geoffrey Cooper, author of *The Cancer Book*, 1993)

1

2000: 'More than one million people in the United States were diagnosed with cancer in 1990. Cancer (in the US) claims more than 500,000 lives every year. Basing its estimates on statistics, the American Cancer Society predicts that by the year 2000, about one out of every two people will develop the disease.' (Dr I. William Lane and Linda Comac, authors of *Sharks Don't Get Cancer*, 1992)

I hope those figures got your attention, because they certainly got mine. For some, they are merely impersonal abstractions with little personal relevance. But there are those whose experience of cancer's insistent onward march is more traumatic: 'Cancer, and cancer, and cancer. My mother, my father, my wife. I wonder who is next in the queue?' (C. S. Lewis)

Cancer is now the cause of nearly a third of all deaths in Western industrialised countries – up from about twenty per cent not much more than a decade ago. And it is not just because people are living longer – actually we aren't! The life expectancy of a forty-five-year-old person hasn't changed significantly in the last hundred years. In 1870, he or she could expect to live to the age of seventy to seventy-five. Now, he or she can expect to live to between seventy-five and eighty. If average life expectancy appears to have increased by great leaps in that time, it is because there are fewer diseases killing children – and fewer women are dying in childbirth. So the argument that there's more cancer because people are living longer is not a very good one. Overall cancer incidence is increasing at every age level. In 1995, for example, more women of forty had breast cancer than they did in 1955.

Until recently, cancer was a taboo word. Fortunately, it has now come out of the closet. It is no longer seen as an automatic death sentence. The good news is that people with cancer are, according to statistics, living longer, and that forty to fifty per cent of those diagnosed with cancer do not die of the disease. The bad news is that the statistics cannot be trusted, for reasons that will be explained later in this book.

The fact is, more and more people are developing cancer

2

and overall death rates for most cancers have not changed in decades. Some have declined for reasons unknown, while some are increasing at an enormous rate – lung cancer being the prime example. Unfortunately, the cancer research industry is no closer to finding an acceptable cure than it was thirty years ago. On the other hand, the alternative/complementary approaches to cancer are looking much more interesting.

For those of us who do not (yet?) have cancer, two questions pose themselves.

1. Is there any way that I can reduce my chances of getting cancer?
2. If I do get cancer, what is the best way to ensure that I am one of the forty to fifty per cent who do not die from the disease within five years – perhaps even one of the twenty-five to thirty per cent who do not die of the disease at all?

This book is my attempt to answer these questions.

How to improve your chances of not getting cancer

The quick answer is to stop smoking – one in two smokers dies from a smoking-related disease; reduce dietary fat to not more than thirty per cent of total calories (but note that very low fat diets are also associated with some cancer risks – a median fat diet is optimal); eat more fibre; take more exercise; and don't get infected with human papillomaviruses (these are associated with genital warts, *not* genital herpes), which are strongly implicated in cervical, anal and penile cancers.

Alcohol, the other major vice, does not appear to be measurably carcinogenic on its own, unless taken in liver-damaging doses – but evidence suggests that it can speed the passage of other carcinogens into the cells. For heavy drinking heavy smokers this is bad news. Also, avoid exposure to environmental chemical pollutants.

That's the official word on prevention in a nutshell. Change the way you live, to maximise your chances of living a longer, cancer-free life. That's your responsibility – no-one else's. As you read this book, you will come across a number

3

of additional precautions that may very well boost your chances of not getting cancer.

Being prepared for cancer

The statistics demonstrate beyond a shadow of doubt that something very frightening is happening. It may not be exploding as fast as AIDS, but the cancer spectre is much larger and affects many more people. And dying of cancer is a painful, debilitating, traumatic and traumatising experience.

Confronted with my wife's newly diagnosed illness, I discovered I knew nothing at all about cancer. Cancer was just a word. I talked to my friends, supposedly bright, literate and highly educated. None of them knew anything worth a damn about cancer or its treatments. Here is a disease that is going to kill one in two of us within the foreseeable future and we knew nothing about it. Nor were we doing anything about it. We had simply blinkered ourselves to reality. We didn't do it consciously, but we were doing it – like lambs to the slaughter.

Why isn't everyone panicking?

I think part of the reason is that it is all happening so slowly. There is an experiment that went as follows. A number of frogs were put into a shallow pan containing scalding hot water. Without exception, they immediately leapt out. A number of other frogs were placed in a similar pan, containing water at room temperature. This water was ever so gradually heated. The water heated up, but the frogs didn't move. They all eventually died of heat shock.

The moral of this experiment is that when something is gradual, it slips under our genetically primed warning systems that are geared to protect us against sudden or gross changes in our environment. We become habituated. The slow, creeping increase in cancer and heart disease has slipped through more or less unannounced. Yes, there have been stories in the press, but the sense of urgency is entirely missing. We may be able to perceive it intellectually, yet we are not emotionally alerted. Our fight or flight systems are not switched on. There's no adrenaline. There's no panic. We continue to live as we have always lived. One of the purposes of this book is to trigger a little adrenaline.

4

'Why should I read this book before I get cancer?'

The answer is simple. If you don't read this book, you will almost certainly be a victim, because when confronted with a diagnosis of cancer, you will make choices that you may later regret. You need to be informed that there is a medical war out there, with major disagreements as to how cancer should be treated. You need to know what the issues are. You need to understand what the arguments and the options are. You need to read this while your mind is clear and unworried.

Imagine your doctor were to tell you today that you had cancer. How would you react? Many people have had the following experience. One day a doctor does a test and the result comes back positive. Oh my God! It's CANCER! The doctor puts on a very grave face and says he has to put you in hospital. He recommends surgery, followed by radiotherapy and chemotherapy. There's no time to think. The doctor says the greatest urgency is required: 'The quicker we open you up, the quicker we can deal with this thing before it gets too big, before it spreads.' Oh my God! It's going to spread! Panic! There's no time to think.

There's no time to make a reasoned assessment of all the options, no time even to think up the questions you know you should be asking. And anyway, the doctor knows what's best. Before you know it, you've been cut open and then blasted with rads; your hair has fallen out; maybe half your rectum has been cut off and you have to carry a plastic bag around with you for the rest of your life. Then you come across this book. Only then do you see the range of options that are available. And yes, it seems that for some cancers established medicine does seem to have made good progress. And yes, a number of alternative therapies do seem to offer attractive – viable – alternatives.

The fact is, you need to know what you're going to do *before* you get cancer. If you don't, you may find that things are done to you that in retrospect you would rather hadn't been. Only if the patient is forewarned about the battle and where the lines are drawn can he or she be in a position to make the right choices. These are the choices each patient makes for him or herself based on the best available information. Unfortunately, most books on cancer cure concentrate on selling individual cures, rather than raising the issues or on informing the patient before he or she becomes a patient of other possible cures. This book attempts to correct that situation. It is not about acceptance. It is about fighting.

You – not your doctor – are responsible for your decisions

Here is the opinion of a qualified doctor, Dr Eugene D. Robin: 'The doctor's opinion is not infallible. You, the patient, have the highest stake in the decision – the most to gain and the most to lose. You, the patient, are the one to decide what constitutes a happy and productive life. Don't let your doctor, however well intentioned, usurp this right.' Dr Robin's point is that if you don't want an operation because you don't want to live with its consequences, then it is your right not to have that operation.

To make any decision, you need to understand the range of available options. That is what this book aims to provide. You also need to consider the options coolly. The moment you are diagnosed is not the time to start informing yourself about cancer. The time is now. Read this book. Then keep it on your shelf so that when you, or a member of your family, or a friend, a colleague, a neighbour, gets cancer – as they assuredly will – then you will have immediate access to information.

Foreword for people who have cancer

You have cancer. That, of course, is not good news. But there is a very good chance that you will survive it.

Hope is important
More than anything else, your hope that you will be cured will be a significant factor in extending your life and recovering from cancer. Focus your thoughts on that hope and strengthen it in every way you can. You will live! If you find it difficult to think positively about the outcome of your disease, then find a counsellor to talk to, and/or a group of fellow patients – and read the last half of this book, which focuses on non-orthodox therapies. People have recovered from terminal cancer! People have had instantaneous cures! This is all documented. There is every reason for hope. If you don't believe me, read *Remarkable Recovery* by C. Hirshberg and M. Barasch.

Faith is important
No matter what form of treatment you are undergoing or planning to undergo – whether it is macrobiotic diets or chemotherapy accompanied by bone marrow transplants – make certain of one thing: this is the treatment that you believe in most. Don't let your faith be undermined. If you don't believe in the treatment, then stop now – there is a good chance that it won't work.

Visualise success
Visualisation is a method of putting the body into a state of relaxation, then picturing in the mind the desired state (a cancer-free body) or process (radiation attacking the cancer like golden bullets while leaving the normal cells untouched). Some people cannot picture the required

7

state, but they can put it into words. Repeating the message over and over again, letting the words sink to the deepest levels of consciousness, is also effective. Harness the other senses – smell and taste the destruction of the cancer. Bring in the emotions – hate the cancer, love the body. The more total the visualisation, apparently, the more successful it is.

Secrets are dirty

Don't keep your cancer a secret. Tell everyone you know. Why? Because you will be surprised at the amount of attention and support that you will receive. Yes, OK, some of the people you thought were friends won't know how to react to the news and you may lose them. Never mind. They wouldn't have been able to help anyway.

Another, very important, reason for telling people is that they may have information of value – a doctor who's good, a herb that helped someone, a new discovery that so-and-so's nephew knows all about – or they may be able to help you in some very useful way, such as driving you to appointments, searching for information on the Internet, talking to you about it. If you don't tell people, they can't help. You will also feel better if you aren't always trying to protect your secret.

One person you may wish to talk to is a counsellor. See this person as a healer of the emotional life, as well as a completely neutral advisor whom you can bounce ideas off on the way to clarifying for yourself how you feel. You are going through a very scary, very fearful time, and every source of help should be accessed.

Reducing depression

You may be feeling very low and feel that hope and faith are quite beyond you. Yet it is important to feel as positive as you can. Ask your doctor to recommend an anti-depressant. Some doctors recommend taking large doses of vitamin B complex (up to ten B-50 pills per day); this will give you a good dose of niacin (B3) which, in addition to being a mood lifter, is very good for the liver – an important fact for cancer patients.

Another mood and health lifter is to get as much exercise as you can manage. If movement is difficult, then do regular

8

deep breathing exercises. Pamper yourself with soft aroma-therapy massages. Indulge yourself in lavender oil baths at home. Visit a reflexologist. Sit in the park. And above all else, watch as many comedy films as you can manage. When was the last time you laughed yourself silly at Buster Keaton or the Marx Brothers? Laughter is very good for you. You will learn more about these and other suggestions in Part Three of this book.

Finally, trust yourself
Trust your own judgements: they are what you live and die by. This book is an honest attempt to provide you with choices. But you have to weigh up the information for yourself. How do you feel about it? What makes you most comfortable? If you want radiation and chemotherapy, then don't let anyone argue you out of it. The same goes for vitamin C or hydrogen peroxide treatment – or just doing nothing (yes, surprisingly, that is a reasonable option for which a sensible supporting case can be made out). If you feel the best way of dealing with cancer is to pretend it doesn't exist, then you should know that this is also a life-prolonging strategy.

   You are going to read some uncomfortable and surprising things. You may even get angry. All I can say is: hold on to your seats for an interesting ride.

One more suggestion
While you are reading this book, you may wish to start making useful contacts with those who focus on the needs of cancer patients – not doctors and hospitals. Perhaps the most useful thing you can do is to establish contact with The Wellness Community. This is an American organisation which offers a number of completely free services, including day centres, personal and family counselling, visualisation and relaxation sessions and other educational activities. A useful book on their work – and one that gives useful cancer therapy advice – is Harold Benjamin's *The Wellness Community Guide to Fighting for Recovery from Cancer*. A one-week visit to the neighbourhood of a Wellness Community centre may be very effective in helping to re-orientate yourself to your needs and your illness.[1] A British centre based on this model has been set

9

up in Edinburgh. It is called Maggie's Centre, after its founder, Maggie Keswick.[2]

Another book that is a must for cancer patients is *Fighting Spirit*, edited by Heather Goodare, which is a series of personal records of women who have fought cancer – some successfully, some not.

Foreword for carers of people who have cancer

You are close to someone who has cancer. You have a very important responsibility, one that potentially carries with it a great deal of pain. I want to describe for you a story, in the hope that you can learn from someone else's experience and so avoid some pitfalls

One day, a woman discovers she has cancer. She discusses the options put forward by the doctor with her husband and other members of her family. There seems to be no real choice, so she agrees to undergo exploratory surgery followed by radiation and chemotherapy. At the time of diagnosis, she and her husband know nothing about cancer.

While the woman is coping with her disease and the treatments, the husband feels utterly helpless. He decides he must do something. The only thing he can do is inform himself, so he starts to read what he can find. Soon he finds a book that tells him that surgery could be dangerous for a person with cancer – cancer cells can be released into the bloodstream to circulate around the body. By this time, his wife has already had the surgery, so he decides it is better not to tell her.

Then he reads that radiation can be dangerous in itself, much more dangerous than they have been told, and that it can have the effect of making a tumour more malignant. He is horrified. Should he tell her? He decides that he should. She gets angry with him, because she is feeling very vulnerable and doesn't want to know that what she's doing is useless – or worse, even dangerous. They have an argument, the first of many.

Then he reads that chemotherapy for this particular cancer is virtually useless. Again he tells her, again they have an argument. 'What do you know about it?' she yells at him. He can't answer this question. All he knows is that he has

11

read something that seems to be convincing.

All the husband's attempts to support and help his wife are proving to be worse than useless. Instead of bringing them closer, the cancer is causing them to feel very separate from each other. The more he reads, the more he becomes convinced that alternative approaches are the way to go. The more he urges this view on his wife, the more she clings to the treatments she is receiving. The result is damaging to their relationship – and even more damaging to the wife's health. Within a year of diagnosis, she is dead. We can see that getting information too late may be worse than getting no information at all.

The carer's job is a difficult one, and there are few rules. I have been there and made most of the mistakes it is possible to make. I hope that I can pass on a little of the wisdom I have learnt, so that you can avoid these errors.

The need for information
In an ideal world, people with problems will want access to information about those problems. If you are caring for a cancer patient, your first job is to assess how much information that person wishes to have. If he or she is hungry for information, then scour the libraries and bookshops for books on cancer and healing. As far as you can, share the information you are both reading. Make an adventure of it.

Not everyone wishes to have information
Often the carer is far more aggressive in the search for information than the person with the illness. There are many reasons for this. Whatever the reason, the carer must respect this lack of interest. This is difficult and painful, but it may be that the patient is working on the problem at a different level. Denial does have survival advantages. Doing nothing in the way of treatment may also improve longevity and quality of life. Sometimes the carer is much less aggressive than the cancer patient. Don't be another obstacle that has to be overcome in the search for information and support.

Attitudes change
The carer must constantly assess the situation to see if the person with cancer has had a change of heart about the level

12

or quality of information he or she would like to have. One patient may start out with an aggressive hunger for facts but wilt quickly; another may start off rejecting all suggestions but then, one day, the urge to pick up a book may come. Your job involves being sensitive to these changes and adapting yourself to them.

One book is not enough

This book is an attempt to write the one book that should be enough! However, you need to understand that there are major disagreements in the field of cancer therapy and that these disagreements are fundamental. It is a good idea to read around what is available to see how you feel – and, more importantly, how the person with cancer feels – about the range of options.

And if we disagree?

It is very possible that you and the person with cancer will disagree about how the cancer should be treated. The patient may wish to have surgery, radiation and chemo-therapy topped up with hormone treatment; while you may think that large doses of vitamin C, meditation, psycho-therapy and a juice diet might have better results. Or it might be the other way round. Either way, your job is to say your piece once and once only. The ultimate choice is the cancer patient's. What he or she says goes. Once the course of treatment has been decided upon, then follow it through without questioning it. Your job is to give positive support, no matter what choices are being made and no matter what your feelings about them are.

The power of faith and the importance of hope

It is my belief that the two most important responses to treatment are: faith that the form of treatment chosen is a good one; and hope that it will work. No matter what the treatment is, these two attitudes are all-important. They will move mountains. The power of the mind, as we shall see elsewhere in this book, is great. Hope channels the energy of the mind and body into a ray of life-healing force. Your job is to do everything in your power to encourage these feelings. Questioning the validity of a treatment undermines its potential to be effective. So I say again: once a course of treatment has been decided upon, do not question it. Do nothing to undermine hope and faith.

Your relationship is vital
The person you are caring for is utterly vulnerable. Suddenly the future has become murky and fraught. You are a lifeline. Your relationship makes the present bearable. Do everything you can to nurture it.

Be there at consultations
Doctors may be busy, but the person you are caring for is even busier. For the cancer patient time is suddenly in very short supply – potentially – so the patient's time is far more valuable than any consultant's. Don't stop asking questions until you are satisfied that you understand the answers. Get copies of medical tests. Discuss with the cancer patient what you both want to know before you see the doctor, and what you have learnt afterwards. Make sure you take notes of what is said so you can read them through afterwards carefully. This leaves the patient free to concentrate on their direct contact with the consultant. Get clarifications when you need them. You are the advocate. But do clarify the role the person you are caring for wants you to have – don't dominate, but equally don't sit in the background, unless this is what together you have decided your role is to be. This applies just as much whether you are the patient's partner, another member of the family or a close friend.

Is your relationship part of the problem?
This is a difficult question to ask, and perhaps even more difficult to answer. If there are, or have been, problems between you, this may be the time to confront them. Nagging emotional barriers can hinder healing. Healing the emotions can release very profound energy. Professional personal counselling can very profoundly affect the course of disease, and it also has the power to enhance enjoyment of life. Don't be proud. Don't bottle up your emotions. Counselling is for *both* of you.

Lastly, take care of yourself
You are not perfect. You cannot do everything. There will come a time when you too will need to be cared for by

14

others. From time to time, put your own needs first, so that you do not become depleted of energy. People caring for those close to them who have cancer are at great personal risk of ill-health – including getting cancer. The community nursing resources should be investigated. Hospices should be considered for respite purposes. This is also a good time to take up a hobby or further an interest that can act as a safety valve.

Good luck.

Part One

BASIC FACTS

What is cancer?

It is only when we ask this question that we realise how difficult it is to answer. When my wife Bernadette was diagnosed with cancer, I found myself asking 'What is cancer really?' I was confident that I knew the answer, and then as I groped for some image of cancer, I realised I only knew the word. I didn't know the reality that it applied to. I suddenly found I knew nothing. So what is it?

Two answers
Doctors and other health professionals usually give one of two answers.

1. Cancer is not one disease, but a general name for a group of up to 200 diseases, all of which are characterised by rapid and irregular cell growth. Another characteristic is the spread of the disease from one site to another.
2. Cancer is a disease of the whole body, one of the symptoms of which is rapid and irregular cell growth in one or more sites.

The difference between these two answers is crucial. Is the area of rapidly dividing cells the disease itself or only a symptom of the disease? Is it one disease or 200?

Let's return to the question: what is cancer? How we define the disease affects how we treat it. So we must ask ourselves: is the tumour the disease or is it a symptom of the disease? Do we concentrate on attacking the tumour or do we try to heal the body?

Orthodox modern Western medicine considers the cancerous tumour to be the disease itself. How or why it arose they have no idea. But having arisen, it must be attacked. It must be surgically removed. Or irradiated. Or killed with highly toxic chemicals. Or defeated with the aid of an immunological vaccine. Or a combination of these.

Alternative medicine, on the other hand, posits that the tumour symptom will disappear once the root cause disappears. And the root cause, some say, is the fact that the body as a whole has been poisoned and is not getting the right kind of nutritional and/or natural support. To put it another way, there are those who believe that cancer cells have something wrong with them, that they are deviant, and because of this they must be destroyed. The other view is that cancer cells are essentially normal cells forced to live in and accommodate themselves to an abnormal tissue environment. The problem is not the cells *per se*, but the surrounding environment.

WHO IS RIGHT?
We are so used to right-wrong polarities that it seems easy to ask this question and get a definitive answer. Yet potential patients – and we are all potential patients – must be very wary of taking a one hundred per cent position. Perhaps we need to embrace the question with both hands and suggest that there may be an element of right on each side.

It is certainly true that some people have been diagnosed with cancer, have undergone surgery, with or without radiation and chemotherapy, and have gone on to live long and happy lives. This is true of my own mother, who had breast cancer eleven years ago and who has had no further problem following surgery and radiation treatment. It is also true that what appears to work for one type of cancer will not work for another – and therefore it makes sense to talk of different types of tumour. So on these grounds, we have to accept that the orthodox medical approach has some merit.

It is also undoubtedly true that some people have utterly rejected these therapies and have cured themselves of cancer by doing no more than drinking a particular herbal tea, or even by simply mentally rejecting the disease. One case is that of Dr Benjamin Spock, who in his early eighties was diagnosed as having a bone cancer in his spine. At his age, he had no desire to undertake any burdensome treatment. He also knew that cancers grow slowly in elderly people. He decided, therefore, simply to refuse to believe he had the

20

cancer. A few years later, tests showed that the cancer had gone.

Some people have problems with anecdotal evidence of that sort. I don't. But what often happens in cases like this is that sceptics call into question the original diagnosis: how can we know that he really had cancer? But they don't call into question the cases that respond to orthodox treatments.

What is cancer? In a sense there is no right, objective answer to the question. The answer we choose for ourselves depends on the medical model that we choose to follow. What is important is that we know there *is* a question, and that there is no simple black and white answer.

Before proceeding with the discussion of cancer treatments, let's look at some basic facts.

What is a tumour?

A tumour is a growth that contains both normal and abnormal cells. The abnormal cells divide faster than the normal cells. The rate of division varies. Some tumours grow very slowly, while others are more aggressive. Tumours are not always cancerous. The classic division is between benign and malignant tumours. What do these terms mean?

A benign tumour generally has limited growth potential – though there are cases even today of tumours weighing 13–18kg (30–40 lb) being removed from a person. Most, however, soon stop growing. They do not grow rapidly and they do not destroy normal cells. Another feature is that they do not spread. The technical term for this process of spreading is metastasis. Since the benign tumour does not metastasise, it remains localised in one site. It grows in an orderly fashion, and does not produce serious side-effects unless it is pressing against an organ, like the brain, in a limited space.

By contrast, a malignant tumour will keep on growing relentlessly and does not stay within the normal organ boundaries like other cells do. It is capable of sending particles away from the main tumour, which can then travel to distant parts of the body to develop other tumours. Frighteningly, this can happen many years later.

Malignant cells vary to differing extents from the original cells normal to that tissue. Confusingly, doctors use the

21

term 'undifferentiated' to describe cells that are very different from the normal tissue cell. The reason for this is that normal cells are differentiated (i.e. specialised) according to the tissue they belong to. From time to time, these cells are worn out, die and are replaced. They are replaced from stem cells that do not have a specialised appearance. So when the stem cell produces a new cell, the new cell goes through a series of changes before it can become a differentiated, functioning tissue cell.

It is believed that cancer occurs when something goes wrong with this differentiating process. The earlier in this process the error occurs, the greater the problem. This explains why cancers of the heart and nervous system are extremely rare in adults. These tissues are noted for their very low tissue replacement rate. For this reason, damage to heart and nerve tissue is generally permanent. This also explains why most cancers of the nervous system occur in children – i.e. when nerve tissue is being created.

Tumours are classified according to the type of tissue involved.

- **Carcinomas**: the most common form of cancer, arising from the tissue that divides most often: the surface cells of organs, or the cells that form the linings of the body and its organs; e.g. skin, lung, intestinal, uterine and breast cancers.
- **Sarcomas**: these arise in the muscle and connective tissue. They attack bone and muscle.
- **Myelomas**: these attack the blood plasma cells in the bone marrow.
- **Lymphomas**: lymph is a water-like fluid that bathes and cleanses all the cells of the body. It originates in small, bean-sized nodes and glands. Lymphomas attack these lymph organs.
- **Leukaemia**: cancer of the blood-forming tissue and blood cells characterised by the over-production of white blood cells.

Tumours are also classified according to the stage of their development:

- Stage 1: small tumour with no signs of spread.

22

- Stage 2: some local spreading has occurred.
- Stage 3: more widespread local metastasis is detected.
- Stage 4: the cancer has spread to different sites.

The symptoms of cancer

Unfortunately, it is rare for any symptoms to become evident before a cancer has reached a fairly advanced stage. X-rays, for example, can only detect lumps of about 1 cm (½ inch) in diameter.

The American Cancer Society issues the following warning signs:

- unusual bleeding or discharge from any orifice
- a solid lump
- a sore that doesn't heal
- changes in bowel or bladder habits
- persistent hoarseness or coughing
- indigestion or difficulty in swallowing
- any change in a wart or mole.

Cancer doesn't necessarily kill!

It is not inevitable that a cancer left untreated will proceed to a terminal stage – some cancer tumours simply disappear of their own accord. This is usually associated with a deep-seated change in the emotional life of the patient, but may be connected with placebo cures, or even dietary changes that have been assumed not to be therapeutic. The incidence of this is usually quoted as being anywhere between one in 10,000–40,000, but there is some evidence that it may in fact be much more common.

Other patients appear to be able to live in a static, symbiotic relation with untreated cancer tumours that grow neither bigger nor smaller. Professor Michael Baum of King's College Hospital, London, estimates that thirty per cent of all breast cancers are self-limiting – i.e. they need no treatment at all.

Cancer and pain

Cancer is generally painless – but if you feel pain, don't accept your doctor's opinion that it can't be cancer. If a tumour presses against a nerve or other healthy tissue, it may indeed cause pain. Pain is a subject about which a great deal more could and should be written. It is a subject that divides orthodox doctor and patient profoundly, as the following conversation reveals.

Patient: I have this pain. It goes right across my back from the spine round to the side.

Doctor: Cancer doesn't cause pain.

Patient: (*slightly bewildered by the doctor's reply*) Yes, but I have this pain. I've had it for some time. It is all over here (*indicating the rear pelvic area*).

Doctor: No, the tumour is quite painless.

Patient: (*thoroughly confused*) It's very painful, especially round here (*indicating the hip*).

Doctor: (*impatient at the patient's inability to understand simple facts*) Cancer tumours don't cause pain.

Husband: (*impatient with doctor*) She's telling you she's in pain and that she wants you to do something about it!

In this case, the doctor is focusing only on the cancer, not on the patient's needs. This is a true conversation. The patient was my wife. And in this case the doctor was wrong. The tumour caused pain, because it was rubbing against other tissue or a nerve.

Doctors generally ignore pain because it is a 'broad pathway' – too many possible causes express themselves as pain – and so it does not aid diagnosis. The degree of pain is no help in ascertaining the extent of the problem. Doctors,

24

therefore, are unable to analyse the pain and trace it easily back to its cause. Since it is not part of the problem and not helpful in diagnosing that problem, doctors often ignore it.

Patients, however, need to understand that pain – because it is subjective and cannot be measured objectively – is not a major part of any established medical equation when it comes to making decisions. This is simply a fact.

Terminal pain

Cancer does cause pain when it reaches a terminal stage. This pain is extreme and it is usually managed – if that is the word – with morphine. It is caused when the tumour takes over the body's energy-generating system for the purpose of its own energy requirements – this is the pain of the body's own tissues dying.

There are other ways of managing pain apart from morphine, and anyone suffering chronic pain should investigate the books available on the subject. The problem with morphine is that it can so disorientate patients that they are unable to respond sensibly to the people around them. For the dying person and those people seeking to come to terms with death, this can result in traumatic loss.

The final stage of death by cancer may entail a state of terminal confusion, a state which may not be total. I would guess that terminal confusion is to be found more often in hospitals than at home.

For further information, read the very comprehensive pain control book *You Don't Have to Suffer* by Susan Lang and Richard Patt.

Causes of cancer

Alcohol

As drinking alcohol is considered a vice, it seems obvious that it must be bad for us. The problem for researchers is that alcohol and tobacco abuse seem to go hand-in-hand – alcoholics tend to be heavy smokers, smokers generally enjoy a drink or two. Separating the effects is therefore fraught with experimental difficulties. There appears to be, in excessive quantities and in association with other pollutants, a measurable tendency for alcohol to exacerbate a cancer risk for the lips, mouth and throat.

Against this, it is now generally accepted that alcohol in certain quantities has a beneficial effect on health. The divisive question is: 'At what level of intake does alcohol cease to be beneficial?' Some researchers in Boston claim that two or three glasses of wine a week is the maximum associated with good health in women. This research was based on a study of 121,700 nurses over a nineteen-year period; it suggested that two glasses of wine a day was not as healthy as no wine at all.

A British study of 12,000 doctors between 1978 and 1991 showed that the most healthy were those who drank 8–21 units of alcohol a week, i.e. up to three glasses of wine a day. However, it took around 60 units of alcohol a week before the death rate equalled that of teetotallers. This would allow a bottle of wine plus a nightcap. So does this mean that what's good for men is bad for women? Possibly.

Not all alcohols are equal. Beer is supposed to be good, as it restores the pH of the body to a healthy state. (pH is a means of expressing the balance between acidity and alkalinity.) Red wine is good for reasons to be found in the grape, but spirits are universally frowned upon.

The benefits of alcohol relate, however, not to cancer but

to heart disease. So it is possible that a slight cancer risk is outweighed by greater heart disease benefits. Certainly, rural Greeks who like to drink a glass of red wine with their meal have one of the highest life expectancies in the world. But French men, who are not abstemious, have one of the world's highest cancer rates for men (fifth) – more than double that of French women, who have a far lower incidence (thirty-fifth). Do drinking habits explain this difference? If so, then what do we make of the figures for England and Wales, where men are ten per cent less likely to die of cancer than the French? Do they drink less? Is beer healthier than wine? Or, heretical thought, is the English diet healthier than the French? Some studies suggest that tea drinking protects against cancer.

The answer, of course, may have little to do with dietary factors. Yet diet is known to be a major factor. In the case of stomach cancer, to give another example, the Japanese have a much higher rate than Americans – but third-generation Japanese immigrants to America have the same cancer rates as their white American neighbours.

Cellular adaptation to environmental changes

Some researchers say that large doses of any pollutant for a limited period of time are unlikely to lead to cancer. But even low doses of a pollutant over a *long* period may result in cancerous growths, as the tissue attempts to adapt to the change in its environment. New carpets that have been treated with a variety of chemicals have been implicated as a cancer cause.

Studies have shown that long-term exposure to vehicle exhaust is a definite risk factor. Chemical workers have to be concerned about bladder cancer (from exposure to 4-aminobiphenyl, benzidene and/or naphthylamine), lung cancer (from exposure to Bis, or chloromethyl, ether) and liver cancer (from exposure to vinyl chloride). Having noted that benzene and vinyl chloride are known to be dangerous to chemical workers, how do you feel about the following?

Pollution has also introduced a number of carcinogens into drinking water, including known occupational carcinogens such as benzene and vinyl chloride. However, the amounts of these chemicals in drinking water

27

are very small compared to those in the workplace, and consequently do not seem likely to represent any significant carcinogenic risk. (Cooper, 1993)

Dietary fat and sugar
High dietary fats and sugar are implicated in a number of cancers – but very low-fat diets are too. A median-fat diet is best. High-fat diets are associated with colon cancer, and possibly with breast cancer as well, although this is controversial. Some people suggest that the correlation of sugar intake and breast cancer is much higher than the correlation with high dietary fat. (Studies of mice support the high-fat link with breast cancer.) However, a large-scale study in the US involving 90,000 women failed to find any dietary differences between those who got breast cancer and those who didn't.

Dietary fibre
Low-fibre diets are strongly correlated with high incidences of cancer of the colon and rectum. High fibre is associated with lower colon cancer risk.

Electro-magnetic fields (EMFs)
Electro-magnetic fields have also been implicated as a major cause of cancer. This means that not only is the electrician who works with electrical systems every day at risk, but so is the person who uses an electric blanket and the child who sleeps in a house near a power line. This link has yet to be proved – but evidence is mounting.

One study conducted by the University of North Carolina School of Public Health found that children of mothers who slept with electric blankets developed 250 per cent more brain tumours, seventy per cent more leukaemias and thirty per cent more cancers than those who didn't.

One of the earliest reports on the dangers of EMFs appeared in the *Journal of Occupational Medicine* in 1985. This article reported that deaths in Maryland from various cancers were up to three times higher among electricians, electrical engineers and linesmen than any other occupation.

Since World War Two, we have filled the air with electromagnetic waves. They beam down on our houses through telephone wires, television satellite dishes and radio receivers. Add to this beepers, cellular phones and CB radios. Then there are the electrical coils in the kitchen, electric blankets and overhead power lines. We are dependent on EMF-producing equipment. If EMFs are dangerous, then we have problems. Dr Robert Becker, a world expert in this field, is in no doubt: 'At this time, the scientific evidence is absolutely conclusive: 60-cycle magnetic fields cause human cancer cells to permanently increase their rate of growth by as much as 1600 per cent and to develop more malignant characteristics.'

Free radicals

Free radicals are highly reactive molecular fragments that are hungry for oxygen. If left uncontrolled, they would quickly destroy every living creature as they scavenge for oxygen in the cell walls – so damaging the cells. They cause mutations to the cell's DNA, which can result in cancer. Very little, if anything, is mentioned about them in orthodox medical cancer books. One reason is that the main orthodox anti-cancer weapons *create* free radicals, and the best known means of controlling, or minimising, their effects are through the use of antioxidant vitamins (vitamins A, C and E). Since the use of vitamins is generally decried by proponents of orthodox medicine, the subject of free radicals is an intellectual no-go area.

Gender

Men tend to have a higher risk of getting cancer than women. Each year, for every 100,000 population, between 54.4 (Thailand) and 235.4 (Hungary) men die of cancer. For women, the risk varies from 36.4 (Thailand) to 139.4 (Denmark). In only two countries among the top fifty do women have a higher incidence than men: Ecuador and Mexico. The difference in risk between men and women appears to vary from three per cent (Ecuador) to 127+ per cent (France). The figures quoted are for 1986–88 (*Cancer Journal for Clinicians*, 1993).

Intestinal fluke

A very recent idea by one physiologist is that the intestinal fluke – a common human parasite – which normally needs to complete its life cycle with the help of an external animal host, sometimes, because of changes in the body's chemistry, is forced to complete its cycle in the human liver. The result, it is argued, is cancer (see Clark cure, page 193).

Nitrites in processed foods
Pickled, smoked and cured foods are associated with stomach cancer. They contain large amounts of nitrites, which can be easily converted to a class of highly potent carcinogenic chemicals called nitrosamines. Vitamin C is known to interfere with the formation of these compounds.

Reduced immunity
Although generally accepted, the connection between cancer incidence and lowered immune systems is not absolutely proven. For example, people with AIDS, whose immune systems have completely collapsed, do not have a higher incidence of most cancers. They do have a higher incidence of Karposi's sarcoma – an otherwise rare cancer – lymphomas and cancers of the anal-genital area. These last-named cancers are caused by virus infection through sexual activity – particularly Epstein-Barr virus and the human papillomavirus (HPV), which causes genital warts. But although infection by these viruses is widespread in certain areas of the world, it takes a reduced immune system to allow them to form cancers.

This suggests that a lowered immune system is not a straightforward and automatic cause of cancer.

Smoking
We all know that smoking causes lung cancer, although it cannot be proven. The evidence is statistical: smokers die of lung cancer in much larger numbers than non-smokers. It is also historical: before smoking became a widespread habit, lung cancer was an extremely rare disease.

Stress
Stress is often a precursor of illness, particularly cancer, and is known to result in a lowered immune response. Illness is possibly the only way the body can tell the mind that it needs to make a drastic change. If the lowered immunity is allowed to remain for any length of time, then the chances

of serious illness occurring rise sharply. Often people in stressful circumstances feel trapped.

Trauma
Another cause of cancer appears to be physical or emotional trauma. One early study of this phenomenon, in 1893, found that of 250 patients at the London Cancer Hospital:

> Forty-three gave histories permitting a suspicion of mechanical injuries. Fifteen of the forty-three also described themselves as having undergone much recent trouble. Thirty-two others spoke of hard work and privation. In 156 there had been much immediate antecedent trouble, often in very poignant form, [such] as the loss of a near relative. In nineteen, no causation history could be proved. (A Dr Snow, quoted by Carl Simonton *et al*, 1978)

Viruses
Around one-third of cancers are believed to be caused by viruses. One minority view is that *all* cancers are caused by microbes, which can change shape so that sometimes they appear to be viruses and at other times bacteria.

Causes don't equal results
In most cases of exposure to a carcinogen, there are some, usually a minority, who will get cancer – the others won't. That suggests that the physical and mental health of the person exposed is a key factor. This is an old medical argument, but there is no doubt that the terrain of the body has a key say in whether the seeds of cancer will be able to take root and thrive. If this is the case, maybe we should concentrate our efforts on making sure our basic mental and physical health, our contentment and joy, are not intruded upon by the dark spectre of this disease.

The wider sphere
Cancer is not just a disease, it is an event, one that has an impact on the whole family. In addition to the emotional and psychological impact and the impact on relationships, there are also the physical health implications for the rest of the family.

31

For example, cervical cancer can be caused by a virus, and there is evidence that it can be transmitted sexually. If a man's first wife dies of cervical cancer, his second wife has a four times greater chance of having it. There is also a high correlation between a husband having prostate cancer and a wife having cervical cancer. How many cancers have a virus implication? No-one really knows. One theory is that they are the cause of all cancer. At present, this is a minority view, but history demonstrates that all conventionally accepted truths were once minority views. Naturally, this doesn't mean that all minority views eventually become accepted – just that we cannot dismiss an idea simply because very few people hold it.

A major illness, possibly leading to the death of a family member, also has an impact on the immune systems of close family members. There is a measurable lowering of the immune system and therefore a higher likelihood that others will become ill. And it seems that no member of a family in which there has been cancer should have a vaccination. The family should also review the family environment, way of life and dietary habits to see if they can make changes.

Incidence of cancer

Epidemiological studies show that cancer incidence varies greatly from country to country, being low in the Third World and increasingly high in the West. Those who suggest that cancer is also a disease of the spirit need only point to Hungary – the country with the worst cancer rate also has the world's highest suicide rate.

Cancer incidence also varies widely from area to area within a country. Anyone seeking to explore this subject should consult *The Atlas of Cancer Incidence in England and Wales 1968–1985*. Here the reader will find that in Leicestershire, breast cancer in women over forty-five is more than twenty per cent higher than the national average; while in Cumbria, it is more than twenty per cent lower than average. Women in Cumbria should not pat themselves on the back, however. Incidence of malignant melanoma among Cumbrian females is more than fifty per cent higher than average, while just across the Pennines in Durham, incidence is more than thirty per cent lower than average. Curiously, the incidence of malignant melanoma among

Cumbrian men is twenty to thirty-five per cent lower than average.

How can we explain these variations? As Dr Gordon McVie, scientific director of the Cancer Research Campaign, was quoted as saying in the *Independent* on 25 March 1994: 'The difference is far too big to be explained by genes. We have to take a look at diet, at excess calories. It may be that diet is linked in a very complicated way.'

This kind of research reveals that seventy to ninety per cent of cancers relate to lifestyle and environmental factors – only five to ten per cent is gene related. Such research is clearly valuable, because prevention is better than cure. A person who doesn't get cancer doesn't have to be treated with expensive, painful and potentially health-devastating methods.

You and your doctor

As we shall see in later chapters, the patient who is passive in the face of treatment, assigning responsibility to the doctor for achieving health and recovery, is less likely to survive than the person who actively participates in the recovery programme. It will help patients achieve some control if they understand the subtleties of some of the language the doctor may use in discussing cancer treatments.

THE LANGUAGE OF CANCER

Doctors use a variety of words to measure success, and it is important to understand what is meant by the expressions defined in the chart that follows.

Measures of Success

Response Rate	This indicates the number of patients for whom the cancer shrank more than fifty per cent after treatment. But tumours can quickly return. This measure is meaningless for patients. There is no connection at all between response rate and survival.
1-3–5-10-Year Survival Rate	This means exactly what it says: the percentage of patients who were treated have survived for the period indicated. Short- and medium-term survival rates are highly suspect, as they are skewed by improvements in diagnosis. If cancers are found earlier, the survival rates will apparently go up without any actual improvement in treatment.

Disease-Free Survival	How long the patient survives without any signs of the tumour. Length of life may not be increased in any way, even with increased disease-free survival.
Regression/Partial Remission	The tumour has grown smaller.
Complete Remission	Complete disappearance of cancer tumours for a significant period. This sounds less permanent than a cure and usually is.
Cure	Doctors don't often use this word. If yours does, ask what he or she means by it. It may mean no more than five-year survival.

Treatment options

If cancer has been diagnosed, then you will need to talk to your doctor very carefully about treatment options. You have a choice between following orthodox or comple-mentary/alternative treatments. The former are surgery, radiation and chemotherapy, though you can also ask about immunotherapy, anti-angiogenesis therapy, heat therapy and photodynamic therapy. Alternative treatments generally apply to the whole body and so to all cancers. They include a range of options, including diet, supplements and therapies (see Part Three).

For any cancer that has metastasised and where ortho-dox treatments offer poor prognosis, alternative treatments may be preferred, as they are usually not invasive or damaging in the way that orthodox treatments tend to be. Your doctor may well be dismissive of the alternative approach, but bear in mind that this is a professional prejudice, not based on rigorous scientific evaluation. There is a fundamental, ideological dispute between doc-tors, who focus on the tumour to the exclusion of all else, and complementary health practitioners, who focus on the terrain in which the tumour is growing, and aspects of the body's bio-chemistry that may be contributing to the further development of the cancer.

You need to investigate properly the full range of treat-ments available to you – both orthodox and complementary.

Counselling

Many cancer patients have expressed disbelief and anger at the poor quality of the medical counselling they are provided with. It is not uncommon for doctors virtually to order patients to undergo certain procedures. Like the rest of us, doctors are not perfect, and most of them will have had little or no training in counselling. Do not allow yourself to be coerced into making a decision about which you have reservations; if you need a week to decide, take it, even though the doctor may say something unhelpful like 'That's not in the protocol'. This advice comes direct from the personal experience of cancer patients.

However, many doctors – particularly GPs – are caring and sympathetic towards their patients and fully appreciate the emotional turmoil that a diagnosis of cancer brings. Talk to your GP about how you feel. Both he or she and the specialist cancer unit where you should be referred will be able to tell you about the various support services – both emotional and practical – available.

The consultation

When talking to your doctor, it may be helpful to record the conversation on tape or to have someone with you to take notes. Your objective is to get as full a picture as possible of your situation and the options open to you. Persevere if you feel he or she is being evasive, or fobbing you off with reassurance. The following questions may help you to focus on what you need, or want, to know.

QUESTIONS ABOUT THE CANCER
1. Where exactly is the cancer? Please draw a diagram.
2. What stage is it? (Remember the scale of 1–4; 3–4 indicate metastasis.)
3. Is it aggressive or slow-growing? (If it is the latter, you may have more time to make decisions.)
4. What symptoms can I expect if this cancer progresses?
5. What further investigations do you need to undertake? What risks are attached to these?

QUESTIONS ABOUT PROGNOSIS
1. What percentage of people with my condition can expect to live another five years? Ten years?

2. What separates those who live from those who don't?

QUESTIONS ABOUT TREATMENT
1. What are the treatment options?
2. Where will the treatment be done?
3. Who will be in charge of the treatment? (Insist that any surgery you wish to have is done by specialist cancer surgeons.)
4. Are there any other options about where the treatment is done and who does it?
5. Are the treatments being offered to obtain a cure, remission or response? (See above for definitions of these terms.)
6. Can I have copies of any studies into the value of treatment being proposed?
7. Am I part of a clinical trial for this form of treatment?

QUESTIONS ABOUT SIDE-EFFECTS
1. What side-effects am I likely to suffer from each of the treatment options?
2. What are the worst possible side-effects of each treatment?
3. What permanent disability may occur as a result of each treatment?
4. What support/non-medical help can I have throughout and after treatment?

FURTHER QUESTIONS
1. I want a second opinion. Can I have copies of all my medical tests and X-rays? (You may wish to have the opinion of alternative doctors in the United States.)[3]
2. I wish to speak to a specialist oncologist (cancer doctor) about my case – who can I see? (This is if you are not already being seen by one.)

You can talk to your GP about whatever orthodox and complementary/alternative treatments you are interested in, to find out what help he or she can provide. Can the GP prescribe vitamin and mineral supplements, iscador, injections of zinc and magnesium ascorbates, and so on? If the answer is no, and these are some of the treatment options you wish to pursue, change doctors.

Getting a second opinion

There are two very good reasons for seeking a second opinion.

Firstly, many oncologists are involved in ongoing clinical trials, and patients may be recommended a treatment that happens to relate to a current trial – which the specialist may be working on – of a procedure. Patients may not always be informed of this. Patients who are being rushed into a particular course of treatment should be particularly cautious. A second opinion from another source should clarify any possible conflict of this kind.

Secondly, although treatment will ideally be formulated by a team of doctors from different specialities, there may be differences of opinion between those with a medical, surgical or radiological background. The patient should be clear about the pros and cons of the various options before making any decision.

Can we trust cancer statistics?

Looking on the bright side, it is possible to conjure up figures that show significant progress in the battle against cancer. The National Cancer Institute publishes a chart of five-year Relative Survival Rates. The US figures up to 1989 for the top ten killers are given below. (These figures apply to the white population. Figures for blacks are significantly worse, though still showing improvements.)

Five-Year Relative Survival Rates

	1960–63 %	1970–73 %	1983–89 %
Melanoma	60	68	84
Oral	45	43	54
Lung	8	10	13
Breast	63	68	81
Cervix	58	64	69
Pancreas	1	2	3
Leukemia	14	22	39
Liver	2	3	6
Ovary	32	36	40
Colon/Rectum	43	49	60
Prostate	50	63	79
Bladder	53	61	80
Esophagus	4	4	10
Stomach	11	13	17

These figures show clear improvement. So what's the problem? The answer is that five-year survival does not amount to cure.

The incidence of cancer depends upon accurate diagnosis. Improved screening programmes tend to raise incidence figures, because they lead to the detection of many 'early cancers' which either are not cancers, or are cancers which would resolve themselves without treatment; or they find cancers earlier than they would otherwise. Again, with no improvement in treatment, these will have a major impact on official survival figures, as we can see from the following example. Take two men aged sixty-five. One is diagnosed as having prostate cancer and starts treatment. The other is not diagnosed till he is seventy. Both could die at seventy-two, since early treatment may not affect mortality. The first has an apparent survival rate of seven years, the second only two.

Statistics also cannot tell us what any individual's likelihood of recovery will be. If we discover that we have a cancer from which there is a fifty per cent chance that we will die within five years, some people will become very depressed; others will interpret this to mean that there is a fifty per cent chance that they will live longer than five years. Both are correct, but the second patient has the better prognosis.

And what, in fact, does the original statement mean? Is the figure an average (calculated by taking the life-spans of a large sample of patients and dividing by the number of patients)? This is normally how we interpret the figure, but almost certainly this is not what it is. The figure is probably a median (calculated by determining the point of time where half the sample have died). A median-type calculation can say nothing of interest about the fates of those who live longer than five years – all of whom, for the sake of this argument, could live another twenty years without affecting the median calculation. Imagine a group where half the people died before six months and the other half lived ten years. The doctors could present you with the gloomy picture that you have only a fifty per cent chance of living for six months!

Even if the five-year survival rate is only ten per cent, the positive patient will see that this percentage survive somehow. Statistics demonstrate this clearly. The question is: how do they do it? Unfortunately, it cannot yet be answered, because very little research is done on survival.

40

Cures for cancer?

Some cancers are fast growing, others are slow growing. Some stop of their own accord. Others stop after some form of treatment, and still others resist all forms of treatment.

The harsh reality is that between 1930 and 1990, in the US, for men only two cancers actually declined in incidence: stomach cancer has dropped from thirty-eight to seven per 100,000 men and liver cancer has dropped by fifty to sixty-five per cent and now kills only about five per 100,000 men a year. For women, there have been significant improvements in cancer of the uterus, stomach and liver, and some improvement in colon and rectal cancer.

The problem for orthodox medicine is that none of these improvements are recent. There are no sudden drops to show where improvements in surgery, radiation and chemotherapy kicked in. The graphs show long-term trends. More significantly, they show that for many cancers there has either been no change at all or a slow but steady increase in death rates. Prostate deaths have nearly doubled – as have deaths from cancer of the pancreas and leukaemia. And lung cancer deaths have gone through the roof.

Yet there is another way to look at the subject. Cancers are never cured – even when they appear to have gone. The potential for cancer is always there, lurking in the microscopic depths of the body – it can never be said to have been one hundred per cent beaten.

Even talking about winning a war against cancer can conjure up quite the wrong image to some. Hazel Thornton, who was diagnosed in 1991 as having breast cancer, should have the last word:

Whilst I believe that attitude is crucially important in coming to terms with a life-threatening disease so that

41

one may live one's life fruitfully and in tranquillity, I cannot accept that one can say at any given moment that one has 'beaten' the illness. I hope that I am in a state of truce with my body's inefficiencies, rather than waging war with it. (Personal communication, December 1995)

Part Two

THE ORTHODOX APPROACH
TO CANCER TREATMENT

Testing for cancer

The first step in any approach to cancer – as with any disease – is diagnosis. This may occur at a routine physical examination or, more likely, be the result of the patient noticing some bodily changes. Blood tests that will include both non-specific or specific tests may follow: non-specific tests will examine such things as blood counts, calcium or uric acid levels; specific tests will look for tumour markers, chemicals that are produced by various types of tumour. 'Breast, lung and bowel tumors, for example, produce a protein called the carcinoembryonic antigen (CEA). If a very high CEA level is found, then a tumor is assumed to be present until proved otherwise. Similarly, prostate cancers and many cancers of the testicles and ovaries produce known chemicals.' (Dollinger, Rosenbaum and Cable, 1994)

Other laboratory tests will determine whether there is blood in the urine or faeces. Then there are imaging techniques, using X-rays or scanners to see into the body. Or there are ways of achieving direct visual access to parts of the body with specially constructed telescopes, such as the bronchoscope (lungs), cytoscope (bladder), colposcope (cervix), etc. The general name for these kinds of tests is endoscopy – Latin for 'looking at the insides'.

Cytological tests study the cells that have been removed from the body. The Pap smear for cervical cell analysis is the most common of these. Often cells have to be removed through a surgical procedure called biopsy – the removal of cells from the site of a suspected tumour for examination.

Problems with tests

When your doctor says: 'I'm sure there is nothing to worry about, but we'll just do some tests to make sure,' it all

45

sounds very reassuring; and when doctors recommend regular check-ups, the reasoning seems sound. But there are hidden problems.

Let's take the Pap smear, that involves scraping and brushing the inside of the womb to obtain cells for analysis. The removed cells are put on slides, stained with dyes and examined with a microscope. The cytologist will look for the characteristic appearance of malignant or pre-malignant cells. A pathologist should also examine the slides and either diagnose cancer or report a strong suspicion of pre-cancerous cells. According to the orthodox medical establishment, all women over eighteen, or when sexually active, should have a Pap smear test every year or every one to three years after three normal yearly examinations.

Other doctors disagree vehemently with this suggestion: 'Many excellent organisations such as the National Cancer Institute endorse periodic or annual Pap smears for cervical cancer. But neither the opinions of the numerous societies nor of the experts are based on any *acceptable* [author's italics] clinical trial of the risks versus benefits of Pap smear.' (Eugene D. Robin, 1984)

The Pap smear is one of the most widely used of all cancer tests, and in Dr Robin's view the dependency on this test is dangerous. First, there is the risk of the false positive. As a result, a woman may believe she has cervical cancer when she hasn't. Or the reverse, where there is the false negative – a woman is told she doesn't have cancer when she does. Highly qualified specialists study the slides and the cancerous cells have a 'characteristic shape', so how do mistakes happen?

Pap smears require interpretation. Different doctors examining the same specimen under the microscope will vary widely in their opinions. In one study, quoted by Dr Robin, ten experts disagreed about the presence or absence of cancer cells in about forty per cent of the specimens. One reason for this confusion is a non-cancerous state called dysplasia, which occurs in the cells of the cervix and may be difficult or impossible to distinguish from CIS – carcinoma in situ – a form of cancer, or pre-cancer, where the cells remain localised. CIS does not necessarily become invasive cervical cancer (ICC).

Abnormal cells can also appear in the Pap smear as a

result of fungal infections, changes in the metabolic state of the subject, or for other reasons. As Dr Robin remarks: 'The possibility of finding in the Pap smear abnormal non-cancerous cells that can be mistaken for cancer is substantial.' The standard surgical response to a positive Pap smear is often quickly to perform a hysterectomy. Often, the removed uterus will show no signs of cancer. Similarly, women have been found to have invasive cervical cancer shortly after a negative result. The number of false positives and false negatives amount to over thirty per cent of all test results.

The problem for people with false positives is that they may undergo cancer treatment – surgery, radiation and chemotherapy – unnecessarily, from which they may suffer permanent damage or even death. According to Dr Robin, the false negative is a lesser problem than the false positive. His reasoning is that ICC is generally a slow-growing cancer. A woman of thirty-five diagnosed with ICC should live on average for another thirty years. However, a person who dies from the indicated surgery – abdominal or vaginal hysterectomy – will die immediately (his estimate is that two women die for every 1,000 hysterectomies performed; 350 in every 1,000 will have serious complications). Radiation, another response the orthodox doctor may resort to, may cause atrophy of the upper vagina and vaginal scarring, as a result of which the woman will find it painful or impossible to continue normal sexual relations.

Dr Robin seems to be arguing that there is a very good argument in favour of doing nothing in the case of cervical cancer. Let nature take its course. Whatever your views on this conclusion, one thing has emerged: the Pap smear is seriously flawed as a test. It is less so, apparently, when other clear signs of cervical problems exist, e.g. bleeding. Any woman who suffers vaginal bleeding and gets one negative Pap smear should have an immediate re-test; and a further one if necessary.

WHAT ARE THE IMPLICATIONS?
This examination of the Pap smear raises one of the key issues relating to tests. Most tests are not one hundred per cent accurate. When they fail, they do so in two ways: the false positive and false negative, as described.

Very few medical tests are clinically tested – subjected to rigorous scientific assessment – so the failure rate is not obvious. What this means is that a certain percentage of people get the wrong results. The more people who are tested, the more will be given the wrong results. Many doctors, therefore, question whether having annual tests is wise. Why have a test when there are no symptoms? The result of mass testing must be large numbers of people with false positives and false negatives.

Furthermore, it is becoming increasingly understood that people are different. Most tests assume a norm. Variance from that norm indicates, for the doctor, problems. But for every metabolic process there is a wide spectrum of functioning, or performance. What is normal for one person may be abnormal for another. For example, the cyclist Miguel Indurrain has a resting heart rate of twenty-eight beats per minute. The norm is supposed to be in the region of sixty.

Some tests should be avoided because they are unsafe. More than one overweight man has died while having his heart checked on a running treadmill. Some tests require the inspection or removal of tissue in an operating theatre – all such tests have what professionals refer to as a morbidity factor – a possibility of permanent injury.

A test should only be done if it is likely to lead to a treatment. There is no point in discovering that something exists for which there is no known treatment. This is well illustrated by the following personal story. I know a man whose chest X-ray indicated that there was a possibility something was seriously wrong with his lungs. 'These shadows could be old tubercular scars or it could mean lung cancer,' the doctor told him. 'If it's cancer, I can only give you a few weeks or months to live. The only way I'll know for sure is by going in and having a look.' Amazingly, that is what my friend did. The result was painful and expensive surgery that showed there was no problem. I had to laugh when I heard this. 'Why didn't you just wait to see if you were still alive in six months' time?' I asked.

BIOPSIES
A biopsy is the test to see whether a lump is malignant or non-malignant. This information is obtained by cutting out

a small section of the lump and analysing the cells. There are two problems with biopsies – apart from that of interpreting the results. One objection is that they can irritate the lump and so transform it into a malignant tumour. The other objection to cutting a tumour (incisional biopsy, where fine needle aspiration involves removal of part of the internal tissue of a tumour) is that cancerous cells may be released into the bloodstream, so facilitating the spread of the cancer throughout the body. This risk is reduced where the whole tumour is removed for a biopsy – excisional biopsy.

MAMMOGRAMS

Supporters of mammograms suggest that annual breast checks can lead to a twenty-five to thirty per cent reduction in mortality from breast cancer over a period of twenty years for women aged over fifty. A study from the University of British Columbia, reported in *The Lancet* in 1995, found no evidence to support these figures; the recommendations were that mass mammography should be stopped, as it does more harm than good.

Mammograms have a very high rate of false positives – over eighty per cent. Indeed, one Canadian study found that only one in fourteen women diagnosed with a possible cancer actually had a malignant tumour. Women with such false positive results from the test are then likely to have unnecessary surgical and other treatments. This is in part because there is a relatively benign form of breast cancer, ductal carcinoma in situ, which in most cases will not harm the woman who has it, but which is usually treated as aggressively as other more malignant forms of the disease.

There are also disturbing indications that mammograms may not be entirely safe. There is a slight risk – estimated at one per cent – that the X-rays themselves may cause cancer. Supporters of the test point out that X-ray doses used in mammograms are one-tenth of those used twenty-five years ago, and that any risk is minimal. However, one per cent of women have a gene, the ataxia telangiectasia gene, which makes them highly sensitive to radiation. Dr Michael Swift, chief of medical genetics at North Carolina University, estimates that up to five per cent of US breast cancer cases diagnosed each year are the result of mammograms.

In addition, mammograms cause trauma to the breast tissue, as the breasts are forcibly pressed, generally causing pain. And if there is a malignant cyst in the breast, such a process may speed up its development by agitating it. Needle biopsies into suspected tumours cause problems for at least a quarter of the women undergoing the procedure – pain, scars, development of lumps and even lung punctures.

Studies in Canada, Sweden and the US have shown that women who had regular screenings for over ten years had one third more breast cancers than women who had not been screened. The Canadian study showed that a third more women in the screened group died of cancer.

In conclusion, there is no proof that mammograms are beneficial, and there are some disturbing indications that they may not be.

TESTING FOR PROSTATE CANCER

For men, an equally frightening can of worms has been opened by the discovery that prostate cancer incidence is very high. The longer you live, the more likely it is that you have got it. But the simple fact is, most prostate cancer is very slow growing and not aggressively metastatic. You can live a long time with a cancer of this type and not even know it. So, the question is: who cares? There is no point in testing for something that is almost certainly present. The problem, unfortunately, is that some cases of prostate cancer *are* aggressively metastatic.

Alternative therapists say that the herb saw palmetto has a very beneficial effect on the prostate. So it seems to make sense for men over fifty to assume they have the disease, and to be informed about maintaining their general immune system. Of course, once prostate cancer testing becomes standard practice, there will suddenly be a huge increase in prostate cancer with good survivability. These are going to skew overall cancer statistics in a way that will look good, but not be very meaningful.

TEST RESULTS

Finally, another problem rarely mentioned is the reporting of test results. Often this is done by a nurse to the patient over the phone. In my own case, my wife died because she accepted over the phone that the results were negative. If she had read the test report, she would have seen the comment that indicated something was not one hundred per cent right. She would have had a re-test.

So, whenever you have a test, make sure you read the results yourself on the original test result form, and get a copy for your own medical file at home. Be happy to pay any photocopying fees. A good doctor will welcome this as a sign that you are willing to take responsibility for your own health and well-being.

Surgery

To put cancer surgery into perspective, it is worth looking at its history. Surgery was known to the ancients, but was expressly condemned for cancer. Hippocrates' famous comment was: 'It is better not to apply any treatment in cases of occult cancer; for, if treated, the patients die quickly; but if not treated, they hold out for a long time. ('Occult' means hidden.) Here is the argument for doing nothing, a conclusion supported by some modern medical statisticians.

In Europe, medical practitioners between the twelfth and nineteenth centuries repudiated the use of any kind of surgery, leaving it to barbers to perform. Without asepsis or anaesthetics, it was cruel and generally unsuccessful. The great Swiss doctor, Paracelsus (1493–1541), said: 'It should be forbidden and severely punished to remove cancer by cutting, burning, cautery and other fiendish tortures. It is from nature that the disease arises and from nature comes the cure.' So, doctors 600 years ago were able to talk of curing cancer. It was also their combined experience of the disease that surgery was the wrong approach. Now it is considered the standard approach – and natural cures are considered beyond the pale.

It was only with the discovery of asepsis and anaesthetics that surgery, against much opposition, became accepted. The first recorded surgical cure for a cancer was in 1809, when a 10 kg (22 lb) ovarian tumour was removed from a patient who went on to live a further thirty years. Though whether this should be called a cure is a moot point – the tumour was clearly benign.

Since then, surgical procedures and technology have improved by leaps and bounds. There is no doubt that for cases of severe physical trauma, surgery is essential if many victims are to survive. Surgery also offers wonderful gifts to

52

children born with birth defects, such as hare-lips. But cancer is not a severe physical trauma or a physical malformation that needs to be corrected. It matters not what great advances have been made in the area of surgery – the question of its appropriateness in the case of cancer remains contentious; no amount of technological improvement can change this, because the problem relates almost entirely to the nature of cancer rather than to the nature of surgery.

The dangers of surgery

Surgery is an empirical science. Its methods and procedures develop from day to day and are not, generally speaking, subjected to the harsh judgements of clinical trials. It is therefore not a 'proven' form of cancer treatment in any real sense. It is subject to its own fads and fashions. To give an example unconnected with cancer, a Dr Joseph DeLee, in the 1920s, declared natural childbirth to be unnatural and severely traumatising to the baby. He therefore insisted that all babies should be delivered with forceps clamped round the head. Soon this became the standard approach to birth in the United States. The consequence? Infant deaths from birth injuries rose by fifty per cent. It took five years to realise this.

Surgical development still follows this path. The popularity of triple by-pass heart surgery is attributed by some to the charisma of surgeon Dr Denton Cooley, who invited a TV crew into his operating theatre. There is, in chelation therapy, a very viable alternative to the by-pass, but as it doesn't require surgery heart surgeons are unlikely to be interested in promoting it.

Keyhole surgery is another development that has resulted in greater numbers of complications and deaths. All new surgical techniques have to be learnt, and the patient is the classroom where this learning takes place. The pioneers of any new development will have proceeded cautiously and carefully to build up their expertise – but as soon as the new techniques are publicised, the next generation of practitioners believe they can master them speedily. It took almost ten years after its initial development before the Royal College of Surgeons issued guidelines on training in keyhole surgery – until then they ignored the problem. Surgeons jumped on the bandwagon: it was a case of 'see one, do one, teach one', according to one anonymous surgeon quoted in the *Independent*. How many people have suffered as a result?

The simple fact is that surgery is dangerous and results in deaths. What is the combined death rate from all forms of surgery? Recent investigations in Britain suggest that the average surgeon has a patient mortality rate of between two and seven per cent. This is measurably greater among those who have had the least experience. It is better to go to a big hospital than a small local one. It is better not to be in hospital when medical students graduate and relieve their more experienced superiors. Surgeons undertaking fewer than five breast cancer operations a year have a death rate of up to twenty-one per cent. A specialist is always better than a general surgeon.

Not a 'proven' treatment for cancer?
Against this background, we can now take a hard look at cancer surgery. Surgery can be categorised as specific, or localised, when it simply aims to remove the tumour and nothing else. It is called radical when parts of the affected or neighbouring organs or lymph glands are also removed.

SIMPLE SURGERY
The argument for simple surgery to extract a tumour only – e.g. a lumpectomy, in the case of breast cancer – appears to make a degree of sense. As long as metastasis has not occurred and the tumour is accessible and small enough to be removed, the chances, most surgeons say, are reasonably good that surgery will be sufficient treatment: 'Early stage tumors (e.g., carcinomas in situ) that have not yet invaded surrounding normal tissue can be completely removed and are virtually one hundred per cent curable.' (Cooper, 1993)

This, unfortunately, neglects an important point. Cancer tumours are highly individualistic. Just because a tumour is small does not mean it hasn't metastasised; just because it is big does not mean it is going to metastasise. And, in any case, most tumours are relatively far advanced by the time they are detected – even though they may be small. So, it is not obvious before an operation which tumours are best treated by simple surgery and which are not.

Added to this is the question of the surgeon's competence. One US study suggests that even when a tumour

54

appears to be singular and operable, in only fifty per cent of cases is the entire tumour removed. In half the cases some cancerous cells are left to rebuild the tumour. In addition, the cancer tumour may inadvertently be cut, releasing cancerous cells into the bloodstream. The result? A cancer that spreads much more quickly. When this happens, the result is that not only does surgery not cure, it hastens death – just as Hippocrates observed.

Even biopsies – that most frequently performed of minor surgical interventions – are not problem free. This procedure can itself release seed cells into the bloodstream. The more aggressive the malignancy, the more dangerous a biopsy is. In cases of testicular cancer, one of the most aggressive of all cancers, even biopsies should not be performed.

It is also not widely known that a primary tumour in one site, as well as seeding metastases to other sites, may also have the ability to control these metastases in such a way as to prevent them from growing. Once the primary tumour is removed, the means of control is also removed, with the result that each metastasis can blossom into a full-grown tumour in its own right. This is another argument against proceeding automatically with surgery.

RADICAL SURGERY

Radical surgery is almost always worse than useless. It is a desperate, and almost certainly vain, attempt to remove a cancer that has spread by cutting out all the tissue surrounding a tumour – or trying to locate and remove all the metastases of a tumour. With any such major surgery, the mortality risk must necessarily be greater. For the patient, the pain and suffering are appalling. They may not only be seriously disfigured, lacking in basic bodily functions and weakened, but on top of that their remaining life span may be reduced.

Dr Hardin Jones, Professor of Medical Physics at the University of California, studied the effectiveness of standard cancer therapies. It was his opinion – based on statistical analysis – that there was no relationship between the intensity of treatment and survival rates. Radical surgery, in short, does not improve your statistical chances of full recovery. He is on record as saying: 'Radical surgery does more harm than good.' In fact, he couldn't find any statistical evidence that any kind of 'proven' medical therapy worked: 'The possibility exists that treatment makes the average situation worse.'

One 1949 study on stomach cancer showed that there was no difference in survival rate between those having localised surgery and those who refused. However, survival rates were cut in half when radical surgery was performed.

For most patients, the stated reason for radical surgery will be that the tumour is known to have metastasised – or is assumed to have done so. Once this has happened, there is no knowing where the secondary tumours will appear. The tissue closest to the tumour will not necessarily be the tissue first affected by a new metastasis. The cancer cells may have been borne by the bloodstream to areas of the body far from the original site. Breast tumour cells may grow in lung tissue, or in the bone, or in the kidney – nevertheless it remains a breast cancer cell, identifiable as such under a microscope. Once a tumour is suspected of metastasising, then surgery ceases to be a sensible option: what is the surgeon going to cut out? When will the surgeon finish cutting?

Mastectomy: a special case

The most common form of radical surgery is mastectomy – which involves amputation of the breast, the fat under the skin surrounding the breast, the muscles on the front of the chest that support the breasts and all the fat and lymph nodes in the armpit. This may be done because the cancer already shows signs of spreading, or as a preventative measure to make sure that the cancer tumour doesn't spread.

Amazingly, of those women who survive long term after a mastectomy, five to ten per cent will later find a cancerous nodule on the mastectomy scar. Despite this, in the US, large numbers of mastectomies are performed as a preventative measure. Women are voluntarily having their breasts removed in order to avoid breast cancer. Figures from one New York hospital showed that such prophylactic mastectomies accounted for twenty per cent of the total!

The radical mastectomy itself is done far more often in the US than in Europe, but a modified version is increasingly being used in Britain. There is no evidence that it is effective, and it is considered by many surgeons to be unnecessarily brutal. One US critic of this operation, Dr George Crile, commented: '[Radical mastectomy] seems to have been designed to inflict the maximum possible deformity, disfiguration and disability [on the women who receive it]'. (Quoted in Moss, 1982)

Survival rates for women who have a mastectomy are no greater than for those who have a lumpectomy – about fifty per cent will survive five years. Yet women undergoing breast surgery very often don't know which procedure will be done on them. Sometimes, women undergo mastectomies simply because there is too great a pressure on the radiotherapy unit of their hospital – lumpectomies, in the UK, are often accompanied by radiation. A 1995 *British Medical Journal* review of the effectiveness of lumpectomy versus mastectomy found them equally effective. As for radiation, the review noted: 'It seems that radiotherapy prevented some breast cancer deaths, but caused some other deaths.' Hardly a ringing endorsement.

Not all doctors approve of surgery
Medicine is an arena of contending ideologies. One of these ideologies is the surgeon's creed that the best thing to do with a tumour is to cut it out. This belief has become so dominant that it is now almost unquestioned within the temples of modern medicine – but there are those who disagree.

One hundred years ago, a homeopathic doctor, Dr Compton Burnett, a scathing critic of surgery for cancer, scornfully described the surgical process:

[The woman] was successfully operated on and thoroughly cured thereby of her mammary tumour; nine months later, she was again thoroughly cured of another tumour, by a perfectly successful operation; a few months thereafter she was again successfully operated on for another tumour, and just as she was getting well – she died.

Elsewhere, he remarked: 'Surgeons may think the cutting out and cutting off processes "curing"; I think them a last

57

refuge of helplessness.' Compton Burnett was not alone. Dr Robert Bell, a senior staff member of the Glasgow Hospital for Women, agreed. In 1906, he wrote the following:

> I had been taught that this [surgery] was the only method by which malignant disease could be successfully treated, and, at the time, believed this to be true. But failure after failure following each other, without a single break, inclined me to alter my opinion. The disease invariably recurred with renewed virulence, suffering was intensified, and the life of the patient shortened. That cancer is a curable disease, if its local development is recognised in its early stages, and if rational dietetic and therapeutic measures are adopted and rigidly adhered to, there can be no doubt whatever.

Where has this wisdom gone?

Putting limits on surgery
Whether or not any major organ is removed is a matter for patients, not doctors, to decide – although doctors will try to convince you otherwise. Every patient has the right to say that a procedure may or may not be done on his or her body. Patients undergoing any form of surgery should therefore be very clear in their own minds as to how far they are willing to go. If a woman with suspected breast cancer, for example, is willing to have a lumpectomy but not a radical mastectomy, she needs to write this on the consent form before she signs it.

Unfortunately, legal protection for patients is not as strong as it should be. Doctors are allowed a great deal of leeway as to what they can do in the operating theatre, so it is best to get legal advice.

Surviving surgery
In a particular circumstance, there may be very good reasons why cancer surgery is the preferred orthodox option. In these cases, you should go into the operation with the most positive of thoughts: everything is going to work out fine. Positive thinking helps to boost the immune system. Spend as much time as you can watching funny films and laughing your head off (see page 9 for more details).

Post-operative recovery

After an operation, you can improve your healing in a number of ways that few doctors will be aware of, or advise even if they are aware of them. One is to take very large doses of vitamins C, A and E, starting a week or two before the operation and continuing for a month or so after. Similarly, acidophilus and other friendly bacteria should be taken in capsule form. Smear undiluted lavender essential oil – available at any shop selling aromatherapy oils – on the scars. It is a marvellous healing agent.

Another precaution, especially if surgery is not scheduled for a number of weeks, is to build up a supply of your own blood to be used if necessary. This is to prevent the – admittedly low – possibility of catching hepatitis or HIV from infected blood. The estimated risk of HIV infection in the United States is one in 225,000, while the risk of hepatitis is one in 6,000. Blood transfusion from other donors can also cause problems when there is a reaction to the foreign blood platelets and/or white blood cells – these may cause hives or fevers. The risk of one or other of these is in the region of one in fifteen to twenty.

The psychological effects that can accompany the removal of any limb or organ are not immediately obvious. Careful mental preparation needs to be undertaken. The importance of this is demonstrated by the following sad true story. An eleven-year-old girl was discovered with advanced bone cancer, with the result that her leg had to be amputated. The operation was, it seemed, successful and the doctors were cautiously optimistic. They arranged for an artificial limb to be attached and she was given physiotherapy. Her condition improved and she was released from hospital. The next day she climbed to the roof of the apartment block where she lived and jumped to her death.

Many people who have had less obvious parts of their bodies removed live on in pain and quiet desperation. Surgery should not be an automatic knee-jerk response to cancer.

Radiation

In 1995, radiation had its first centenary. On 22 December 1895, Wilhelm Konrad Roentgen took his wife downstairs to his laboratory cellar and showed her the apparatus he was working on. He asked her to put her hand on a photographic plate. He turned the machine on. There was a brief whirr of electricity. When he developed the plate, his wife was amazed to see the bones of her fingers and hand. His invention caused an immediate wave of interest in scientific circles, and soon thousands of scientists and doctors were experimenting with it. Roentgen could have made millions by patenting the machine, but instead he gave his invention to the world. He also refused to allow the rays to be called Roentgen Rays – instead calling them X-rays, 'X' because so much was unknown about them. When the Nobel prizes were established in 1901, Roentgen was the first to receive the prize for physics.

The wide use of X-rays soon resulted in the first deaths from radiation burns. Still it remained commonly used for a range of purposes. Some shoe shops even installed X-ray machines as a gimmick, so that parents could check if shoes fitted their children. Nowadays, X-rays are largely restricted to medical use, either diagnostic or therapeutic.

Diagnostic and therapeutic radiation
Diagnostic radiation uses very low doses – but even these doses are associated with a number of dangers, the two key ones being: the potential for causing cancer; and the possibility that genetic damage, that may not reveal itself for generations, may be caused. Since diagnostic radiation is used in mammograms, women who have regular check-ups for breast cancer may be exposing themselves to a higher risk than those who do not.

Therapeutic X-rays use far higher doses. It has been argued that these doses are too high to cause the type of cellular damage that can lead to cancer – but medical history contains at least one well-known case which contradicts this assumption. In the 1940s and 1950s, it was common to irradiate the thyroid glands of children who were believed to have a particular thyroid condition. Many of the children later developed cancer of the thyroid. It was only when this connection was made that such irradiation was stopped. Subsequently, it was discovered that the initial thyroid condition itself did not and had never existed – it was a figment of the medical imagination.

Radiation therapy for cancer patients: the official version

The US National Cancer Institute publishes a booklet entitled *Radiation Therapy and You*, which is provided free of charge to anyone seeking information. The reader is assured that radiation is an effective means of treating cancer:

> High doses of radiation can kill cells or keep them from growing and dividing. Although some normal cells are affected by radiation, most normal cells appear to recover more fully from the effects of radiation than do cancer cells. Doctors carefully limit the intensity of the treatments and the area being treated so that the cancer will be affected more than normal tissue.
>
> Radiation therapy is an effective way to treat many kinds of cancer in almost any part of the body. Half of all people with cancer are treated with radiation, and the number of cancer patients who have been cured is rising every day. For many patients, radiation is the only kind of treatment needed. Thousands of people are free of cancer after having radiation treatments alone or in combination with surgery, chemotherapy or biological therapy.

On the question of risk, the booklet advises that there are a number of side-effects: 'Your doctor will not advise you to have any treatment unless the benefits – control of the disease and relief from symptoms – are greater than the

61

known risks. Although it will be many years before scientists know all the possible risks of radiation therapy, they now know it can control cancer.'

The first problem is that the doctor assumes the terminal risk of cancer is one hundred per cent. Any amount of radiation risk, by this standard, would be acceptable. However, this assumption must be qualified. The simple fact is, no-one knows what the natural history of a cancer tumour is. What would the tumour do if left alone? We don't know. This is not an idle question. There are cases where women have lived with untreated breast cancers for years, where they seem to have achieved some form of static balance with the tumours. It is known that cancers are extremely individual – some spread while still diagnostically invisible; others grow large and still do not spread. Some grow quickly, others grow very slowly. Some lead to speedy deaths, others suddenly disappear. We cannot automatically assume that cancer is a fatal condition.

Secondly, the booklet informs us that 'it will be many years before scientists know all the possible risks of radiation therapy'. Medical use of radiation therapy has been in existence for nearly a century, yet the full extent of the risks are not known. This is worrying. It suggests that no-one has looked very carefully at the consequences of radiation, which does not sit well with orthodox medicine's claim to be 'scientific'.

Thirdly, we are given a blanket assurance; 'they [i.e. doctors] now know it can control cancer'. This sounds positive. Yet if radiation is the cure this statement appears to claim, why is cancer still such a big problem? Presumably, some other expression of frequency needs to be added to modify the statement. Nevertheless, the information we are given here about radiation is clearly designed to calm our fears.

What about side-effects? They may, the booklet goes on to inform us, be negligible or serious – but how serious? *The British Medical Association Complete Family Health Encyclopaedia* is also reassuring: 'Normal cells suffer little or no long-term damage [from radiation]. [However] Radiotherapy may produce unpleasant side-effects, including fatigue, nausea and vomiting (for which anti-emetic drugs may be prescribed) and loss of hair from irradiated areas.

Rarely, there may be reddening and blistering of the skin.' This is as much as the average cancer patient is told about radiation and its consequences. Certainly it is very reassuring – especially as the encyclopaedia goes on to say: 'Radiotherapy cures most cancers of the larynx or skin. The cure rate for other types of cancer varies depending on how early the treatment is begun, but the cure rate can be eighty per cent or higher.'

So what's the problem? Eighty per cent cure rate sounds good. Certainly, if there is general agreement that radiation is effective – and the side-effects not too burdensome – then it makes sense to pursue it. A cure is worth a bit of pain. Cancer is a tough nut to crack. Surely it needs a tough hammer to crack it? Indeed, there are those who believe that radiation should be used more, and have a higher profile in cancer management, because, they claim, sixty per cent of all cancers could be cured with radiation therapy. This contrasts with the thirty-three, forty or fifty per cent that various experts say are being cured. Cancers where radiation is supposed to be particularly successful are: cancers of the cervix, testicles, prostate, lymphosarcoma and Hodgkin's disease (a cancer of the lymphatic system).

Radiation therapy: another view

Yet radiation is not without its detractors. We noted that Dr Hardin Jones had little use for radical surgery. His comments on radiation are similarly caustic: 'Most of the time it makes not the slightest difference whether the machine is turned on or not.' We must remember that Hardin Jones was a medical statistician, working with the death rates, not the five- or ten-year survival rates, which, as we have seen, are not to be trusted as they are influenced by a number of factors such as improved screening methods. Another bio-statistician, Dr Irwin Bross, was quoted in 1979 as saying: 'For the situations in which most radiotherapy is given, the chances of curing the patient by radiotherapy are probably about as good as the chances of curing him by laetrile, because the chances of curing any patient in advanced stages of cancer are very poor, regardless of the method employed.' (Quoted by Moss, 1984)

Radiation therapy: a third opinion

Hang on! On the one side, we have a claim of a very high success rate and on the other a claim that its success rate is close to zero. We need a third opinion. Dr Lucien Israel is a highly regarded French oncologist. In his opinion, radiation should be used in the early stages of Hodgkin's disease (he quotes a five-year survival of eighty per cent). He believes it is also very effective in seminomas of the testicles and in cancers of the cervix, prostate and nasopharynx. Yet he admits that these views are tentative and provisional: 'Apart from Hodgkin's disease and lymphosarcoma, there is much disagreement as to its effectiveness – indeed there have been no conclusive trials – and many physicians prefer surgery, despite the mutilation it entails, because it has the advantage of making a clean sweep – total sterilization by radiation often remains problematical.' (Dr Lucien Israel, 1976)

As we see, he is quite blunt in admitting that radiation is not a proven form of treatment. One would have thought that such a 'successful' method of treatment, in medical use for over eight decades, would be in a position to show hard statistics to prove its value. This appears not to be the case.

Those who have seen hard figures – Hardin Jones and Irwin Bross – are not impressed. Another study in 1968, involving 3,000 women with breast cancer and conducted by Dr Bernard Fisher of the University of Pittsburgh, found that those who received radiation after breast cancer surgery fared no better than women who did not receive radiation. (Radiation is used in these circumstances to kill off tumour cells that may have been left in the local area after surgery. That is why, in breast cancer surgery, a lumpectomy is generally followed by a course of radiation treatment. In some countries there is so much pressure on the radiation services that doctors perform full mastectomies instead of lumpectomies – even when the breast tumour is small and a lumpectomy would be sufficient. See Mammograms, page 49.)

Indeed, radiation may not just be useless – it may be dangerous. Some studies have shown that the rate of metastasis may be greater in cases receiving radiation when compared with cases who did not. A study published in *The Lancet* (November 1974) showed that post-operative radiation of breasts actually increased the death rate.

What do the studies say?

Studies suggest that roughly one-third of patients who receive radiation have a response rate – this means the tumour decreases in size by over fifty per cent. How long the tumours respond is not known. These figures relate to the radiation of actual tumours – not the preventative radiation that often accompanies surgery as a 'safeguard' – which, as we have seen, may actually increase the death rate. To repeat, a response does not necessarily indicate any increase in life span. Regrettably, figures for the success of radiation as a form of treatment for cancer are not easily obtained.

Any analysis of the benefits of radiation must distinguish between those patients whose tumour is treated by radiation and those who receive radiation aimed at an area in the body where there might be cancerous cells, but where there is no observable tumour.

Specific problems with radiotherapy

Clearly, empirical observation allows doctors to claim that some cancer tumours do respond to radiation, to the extent that the cancer disappears and does not return for a long time. On this basis, many cancer patients are subjected to radiation therapy, even when no tumour is evident, as a precautionary measure. Whether or not this is justified has not been properly put to the test, though some studies suggest that precautionary use of radiation is *not* justified. But what exactly are the problems with radiotherapy?

1. MAKING TUMOURS MORE AGGRESSIVE

Many cancers, treated by radiotherapy with apparent success, return; when they do so, they are unstoppably aggressive. American Senator Hubert Humphrey's bladder cancer returned three years after being irradiated. No further treatment was able to slow the progress of the disease. In my wife's case, her cervical tumour disappeared after radiation. However, within three months of stopping chemotherapy, five months after completing the radiation treatment, a tumour five inches long was suddenly found to be wrapped round one of her ureters. She was given three months to live and she in fact died two days short of three months later. By that time, the cancer had spread widely in the pelvic area. This happened with a tumour that, because of its initial aggressive nature, was deemed to be likely to respond well to radiation. This effect should be kept in mind by those patients for whom radiation therapy is advised, not as a cure, but as a palliative treatment.

Radiation also makes the tumour impervious to new treatment. Experiments with animals have confirmed this. Mice that have been irradiated do not respond to substances that have a beneficial effect on the cancers of non-irradiated mice. Most cancer patients go through variations of orthodox treatments before considering alternative treatments. In this context, some Mexican alternative therapy clinics are reluctant to treat anyone who has already had radiation or chemotherapy, on the grounds that it is unlikely that any further treatment will succeed but will, instead, negatively affect their own statistics.

2. NON-RESPONSE TO RADIATION

Not all cancers respond well to radiation, and many are resistant to it – lung cancer particularly. Also, any cancer that has already metastasised cannot successfully be treated with radiation – because radiation focuses a beam of ionising radiation at a single spot or area in the body. It is most successful when used to slow down or reduce the size of aggressive tumours – when its success may be, as we have seen, short term.

One of the reasons why radiation is more effective with some tumours than others, and with some cancers than others, has to do with the level of oxygen in the tumour. Oxygen is vital for the success of radiation. Unfortunately, low oxygenation levels are typical of cancer tumours.

Then again, cells can resist the effects of radiation. In all cells – both normal and tumour – there are enzymes that recognise in the DNA chain the parts that have undergone chemical damage. Some of these enzymes cut out the damaged portions, while others sew up the two fragments end to end, maintaining the proper order. The repair is inevitably often imperfect, and the cell will hand on these imperfections when it divides. This is how radiation damage can have effects long after the original cause. The repair is often excellent and the cell behaves as if nothing had happened. Some tumours – of skin, tongue and lips – respond very slowly to radiation treatment, but in these cases the radiation often has good long-term results. In other cases, a tumour may appear to melt away, only to return with greater force. This is true of certain sarcomas, for example.

Radio resistance, as this effect is called, is a major problem, which has led some doctors to give radiation in small, daily doses rather than at intervals of days or weeks. In this way, the cells are given less time to repair themselves. Early evidence suggests that anyone deciding to take radiation should have many sessions on a daily basis rather than fewer sessions at intervals. However, pressure on radiotherapy services can sometimes make this impossible – a case of health service administration procedures impeding possible beneficial medical practice.

When designing a course of radiation, radiotherapists will calculate an overall figure – perhaps 6–8,000 rads – and then divide this into fractions. At each radiotherapy session, the patient will receive a fraction. (In Britain, rads are known as Centi-Grays 'Cgy'.) Low overall doses of radiation will tend to be less damaging than high doses – but also less effective. Radiotherapists need to balance risk against effectiveness. In the US, they tend to opt for lower doses. In Britain, on the other hand, they tend to opt for higher doses. Critics say that this is because, the British legal system being what it is, doctors do not have to worry about being sued and also because success is measured only in terms of positive outcomes (i.e. destruction of the cancer tumour). If a patient's cancer disappears, then this is counted as a success even though the patient him/herself may die or become incapacitated in the process.

What is most surprising, though, is that there are no generally agreed levels for radiation treatment or what constitutes the best regime. This variation has resulted in higher radiation injury rates in the north and south west of England.

3. RADIATION INJURIES
One of the worst consequences of radiation is the injury it can cause. Injury, unfortunately, is not a random, rare and unforeseeable consequence of radiation treatment. It is an inevitable consequence.

We have already read *The British Medical Association*

67

Complete Family Health Encyclopaedia statement that provided the correct dosage of radiation is given, normal cells suffer little or no long-term damage. This statement appears to be intended to give reassurance, rather than to explain the truth. The fundamental fact is that radiation damage to normal tissues is a *necessary* and *inevitable* part of radiotherapy; this is clearly understood by all radiotherapists, but by very few patients. The reasons are as follows.

Each time a tumour is irradiated, thirty-seven per cent of the tumour cells are not affected at all. The next time, thirty-seven per cent of this thirty-seven per cent is not affected – and so it goes on. Unless surrounding tissue is also attacked, it is impossible to eliminate all the malignant cells by radiation alone. From this, we can see that radiotherapy can never succeed on its own if it is aimed only at the tumour. If radiation is used to affect the surrounding tissue, then the likelihood of success increases dramatically. In fact, the success of radiation as a therapeutic tool rises in exact proportion to the amount of damage caused to surrounding tissues. Damage may be discovered very quickly, or not appear for ten or twenty years – and may then not be attributed to the radiation treatment.

'Radiation can cause loss of function of the irradiated tissues. The different organs vary in their vulnerability to this sort of complication. The liver, kidneys and lungs are particularly fragile; the muscles are also susceptible.' (Israel, 1976) This damage may be very mild, or permanently incapacitating or even life-threatening. The fairly recent use of radiation and chemotherapy together has resulted in higher numbers of patients suffering from radiation-induced problems. Some doctors have established a grading for radiation damage:

- Grade 1: minor symptoms which require no treatment.
- Grade 2: symptoms which do not affect performance and can be managed by simple outpatient methods.
- Grade 3: more severe symptoms, altering performance; may have to be admitted for diagnostic procedures or minor surgery.
- Grade 4: prolonged hospitalisation and major surgical intervention.
- Grade 5: fatal complications.

This list clearly tells us that some patients die from their radiation treatment and that for all patients suffering Grade 2, Grade 3 and Grade 4 damage, pain – even extreme pain – and serious discomfort are the norm. How many patients fall into these categories? No-one is saying.

But what exactly is the risk? As we have seen, this is a difficult question to answer, because there is so much variation in therapeutic procedure from one hospital to another, although doctors have begun to state a figure of five per cent of patients undergoing radiation suffering some kind of serious complication.

One group which strongly suspects that the five per cent figure is a gross underestimate is RAGE – Radiotherapy Action Group Exposure. This is a patients' rights group, set up by Vicky Parker, which acts on behalf of people suffering from radiation damage and which organises mutual support groups in the UK for radiation-damaged patients. Their private estimate is that more than ten per cent of people receiving radiotherapy are permanently damaged. This figure will certainly be higher for women who have radiotherapy for cervical cancers, because of the number of organs so close together in the pelvic area which can also be irradiated. In their case, one would suspect a very high morbidity rate.

It is also becoming clear that some people are more sensitive to radiation than others. Different studies indicate that between ten and forty per cent of women may be highly sensitive to radiation – and so will react more seriously to 'normal' radiation doses. But the patient's own potential sensitivity to radiation is not taken into account when designing a course of treatment.

Just how seriously debilitating some of these side-effects and after-effects are can be seen from the following examples. These are the words of one member of RAGE:

'RAGE'. What a good name. It sums up how I felt when I picked up a magazine and chanced upon an article by Linda. I read it over and over again. I just couldn't believe my eyes. First of all I cried a lot and then I felt a blinding rage. They had said I was an unfortunate one-off. How dare they do these things to us in the name of medical science and then compound their mistakes by trying to cover them up?

I had my [internal radiation] in 1989. By 1992, I had lost my bladder, womb, ovaries and half my vagina. I had lost my career and my self-respect. I also almost lost my family, my mind and my sense of humour. 'At least you don't have cancer,' my urologist cheerfully informed me. No, I thought, I don't have a lot of things, like a sex life, or healthy kidneys. Is this the price for not having cancer? I wouldn't have minded so much, but they insisted I didn't have cancer in the first place. Just a few suspicious cells which could turn cancerous if left untreated.

I've decided not to be suicidal any more. Been there, done that! Mind you, watch this space. This is a good day! What do you do when you're strolling around, or sitting chatting to friends, and you feel the tell-tale damp patch seeping through your clothes, and you realise the blasted 'thing' has developed a demonic mind of its own and let you down again. You wear loads of dark patterned, baggy clothes – that's what you do, in the faint hope of disguising your dilemma until you can reach the safety of a loo. (Kath Ridgard, quoted in the RAGE *National Newsletter*, Summer 1994)

A very common effect of radiation is that it damages or kills the body's glands, an important consequence for patients receiving radiation in the neck or head, as the salivary glands can be badly affected. In 1989, Ryan Werthwein, a ten-year-old American boy, was diagnosed with thalamic glioblastoma, a highly malignant brain tumour. He underwent radiation treatment, which proved to be ineffective. 'The radiation burnt out most of Ryan's pituitary gland, stunted his growth, and hurt his mental functioning. We were never told about radiation's possible long-term effects.' (Ryan's mother, Sharon Werthwein, quoted in Walters, 1993)

Radiation of any of the hollow organs – intestine, bladder, ureter, uterus, fallopian tubes and so on – will have the inevitable effect of damaging the mucous membrane which secretes the moisturising substance that protects the inside surfaces of these organs. This damage becomes far more likely when radiation is combined with chemotherapy, because chemotherapeutic agents are designed to attack cells that divide and multiply rapidly, such as the mucous membrane cells.

One form of damage is adhesion, where the cells lining the inside of the intestine become fibrous, tough and rigid. When this happens in the intestine, blockage occurs, requiring urgent surgery to bypass the problem. The destruction of the organ linings is usually followed by erosion, making perforations inevitable. This allows the contents of one organ to leak into another. Damage to the lymph system is another consequence when the pelvic area is irradiated. This results in extremely painful lymphatic swellings, which vary in intensity and duration, and may be permanent.

Blood vessels are also vulnerable, and haemorrhaging can result – even as long as ten years or more later. Damage can occur to the ureters, the tubes linking the kidneys and the bladder, so that they become blocked. Sometimes a straw-like device, called a stent, is forced up to maintain the flow of urine. The problem is known as stenosis. Where stenting doesn't work, and where both ureters are affected, renal failure becomes a possibility.

Radiation also can weaken tissues, so that they fail at a later date. Intestines can rupture, for example:

Eighteen months after the radiotherapy, I started having violent abdominal pains followed by vomiting. Eventually I was in absolute agony. The pain was indescribable. I began to vomit faecal matter and was rushed into hospital. On arrival, the surgeon warned me that I needed life-saving surgery. When I came round from the anaesthetic, the surgeon [informed] me that the radiotherapy had burned my intestines, resulting in the perforation, causing the bowel contents to leak into the peritoneal cavity, resulting in peritonitis. ('Mandy', quoted in the RAGE *National Newsletter*, Summer 1994)

Management of radiation treatment
Mandy and Kath were victims of an iatrogenic episode resulting from experimental use of a new way of delivering radiation. This happened in a number of hospitals in Manchester and elsewhere, using one or both of two new

71

machines – the Hex 2 and the Selectron.*

Women with cervical cancer are generally treated with both external and internal radiation. For many years, the Manchester Radium Pack was the standard form of internal treatment. Generally accepted as safe, it had a morbidity rate of one to two per cent. Women had a small pack inserted in the cervix for two to three days. Unfortunately, for that time, the patient was radioactive, which affected all those visiting or attending to the patient, particularly the nurses.

To solve this problem, they experimented with a new system called the Selectron. This could be controlled from a distance, so that a nurse attending the patient would not be exposed to radiation. It was also programmed to deliver more radiation over a shorter time. This procedure was then used on patients from 1979 to 1987 – even though problems with it had become evident as early as 1982. The exact cause of these problems was not immediately known, because in some cases the adoption of the Selectron was combined with another new external radiation machine, the Hex 2. The use of these machines appears not to have been controlled in any systematic way.

Another reason for using the Selectron was economic. The shorter treatment time – reduced from seventy-two hours to twenty – enabled more patients to be treated with the same equipment. Radiation machines are expensive. The budgets of radiotherapy units are huge. One radiotherapy Linacs model machine costs £500,000 – and the upgrading of radiotherapy equipment for London alone in the years 1993–1998 was expected to cost £13.6 million. Even this sum is recognised as an underestimate. Selectron machines, which remain very much in use, cost £120,000 each.

Such high costs mean continual pressures to find savings. The best way is to increase the dose delivered each time, so that radiation treatments can be shortened. There is disagreement as to whether the design of the Selectron added to the problems caused by the doctors' decision to increase the dose rate. The result is that some 300 women were condemned to a life such as this:

* Iatrogenesis is the term applied to diseases or harmful consequences that are directly caused by doctors or by standard medical practice.

My life is totally controlled by my condition. I'll never have sex, never marry and have kids, never work again. I'm luckier than some though – some of the women are housebound or bedridden. I can go out when I feel better, though I have to carry morphine syrup with me everywhere. The colostomy bag and my urostomy bag have burst when I've been out, so that's a constant worry, and I have to use incontinence pads all the time. I can't start the day until about 2pm and I tire very quickly. I've been in the operating theatre over two dozen times. Doctors say, 'But at least you're still alive.' But this is no life. It's a nightmare. (Vicky Parker of RAGE)

Funds are rarely provided to investigate possible iatrogenic episodes, but one unofficial estimate of this episode is that nearly sixty per cent of the women receiving this treatment up to 1982 subsequently suffered horrific damage to internal organs. Many are believed to have died, though death certificates will generally state other causes of death. Any suggestion that people die as a direct result of medical treatment is contentious. The hospitals involved in this case refuse to this day to have any contact with those patients wishing to have some discussion about it. None of the hospitals concerned have made any clear admission that their radiation practices are to be blamed. It took over ten years to get the issues properly aired, in the 1996 Channel 4 and Panorama programmes on the subject.

How many women have suffered serious consequences from radiotherapy? RAGE has some 2,000 members who have suffered damage – about seventy per cent of these are women treated for cervical cancer. Some doctors openly dismiss these numbers and say that RAGE is exaggerating the problem, but Vicky Parker retorts: 'How can true stories of members be "over the top"?'

The situation doesn't appear to have substantially changed. The Selectron is being used by more and more hospitals and patients are still not being warned of the potential for damage of radiation. 'Unfortunately, the other day we received a letter from a woman who when she asked re safety of her R/T [in 1993] was told "Everything is OK now – the equipment was fine tuned." She now has bowel

problems, i.e. incontinence, and has written to us for help.'
(Vicky Parker, personal communication to the author,
1995)

We should not assume, however, that this was – or rather
is – a one-off, isolated incident. On the contrary, the
constant implementation of technological 'improvements'
will ensure that episodes such as the one described below
are repeated. Radiotherapy textbooks state very clearly that
radiotherapy is an inexact science, in which procedures are
decided upon in an empirical manner – i.e. if it works it
works, and if it doesn't work then tinker with it until it does.
There is wide variance in practice between one centre and
another.

Nor are such profound disabilities confined to radiotherapy of the pelvic area. Women undergoing radiation for
breast cancers are also at risk. Radiation can damage the
brachial plexus, a nerve tissue in a sensitive area, which may
be heavily irradiated in an attempt to kill a breast tumour.
More than 1,000 women are known by RAGE to have
suffered injuries in the brachial plexus. Some have lost the
use of a hand or an arm, some suffer intractable pain, a few
have even had their arms amputated. This problem affects
approximately one per cent of all women irradiated for
breast cancers. Irradiation of the breasts can also have the
following side-effects: fibrous, shrunken breasts, rib fractures, scarring of the lung and heart, nerve damage and
irreversible obliteration of the bone marrow in the field of
irradiation.

Oedema of the lymph gland is another common result of
radiation, and the result is painful swollen limbs. This is an
intractable problem that requires very careful management.
Radiation of the neck, head or throat will almost certainly
result in the destruction of the salivary glands and possibly
the eventual loss of the teeth.

What's the truth?

What is the actual figure for serious complications arising
from the normal use of radiotherapy? No-one knows. Why
not? Because, in the words of the Secretary of State for
Health to Parliament in 1995: 'The Department does not
keep records of people suffering from radiation damage
after radiotherapy and we have no plans to set up a national

74

register.' Hospitals may or may not keep a record of complications that arise – but they do not publicise these.

Side-effects: the full picture

Given these horrendous potential 'side-effects', you would expect to see clearer warnings being given to the public. But even such organisations as BACUP – a respected national UK cancer charity which provides information to patients – say little or nothing of the risks involved. None of the women involved in the trial of the Selectron remembered being informed. 'It was not our practice at that time to inform patients in detail,' said Dr Robert Pointon, of the Christie Hospital in Manchester, where trials of the Selectron were conducted.

Lady Audrey Ironside, who lost the use of an arm because a thirty-session radiotherapy course was shortened to fifteen double-dose sessions, remembers being told very little by her doctors at the Royal Marsden Hospital in London, only that she would only suffer a few temporary side-effects, such as nausea and exhaustion. 'I was told there were no permanent side-effects whatsoever,' she recalled in an interview with the BBC in October 1991. 'I was never warned of the risks of this treatment and the fact that I could be left with a useless arm and in great pain for the rest of my life.'

RAGE publishes its own list of radiation side-effects, culled from its members, in addition to those mentioned in the newsletter extracts above:

Menopausal side-effects / soreness / inflammation / parasthesia (pins and needles, numbness in legs and feet) / pain / rectal bleeding / constant bladder infections / kidney dysfunction / collapse / vomiting / diarrhoea / severe headaches / memory loss / flu-like symptoms / lethargy / adhesions / contractions / depression / blackouts / falling over / feeling bloated / oedema (swelling of hands, face, legs, feet) / anaemia / abscesses / backache / hair loss / tooth decay / loss of teeth / weight loss / memory loss / altered sleeping patterns / lack of sleep / severe pelvic and abdominal pain / vaginal and anal pain / discharge – front and back passage / foul-smelling bleeding / arthritis / osteoporosis (pelvic bone fractures).

75

If it's so dangerous why is it used?

One reason is that doctors assume all cancers will inevitably lead to death. Professor Karol Sikora explains the general case thus: 'For some forms [of cancer], such as cervical cancer, it is the only hope of cure, and without it thousands of women would have died.' But what this neglects to say is that cervical cancer is, generally speaking, very slow growing. Certainly women with this particular cancer can in the early stages afford to spend some time examining alternatives to radiation – such as those suggested in Part Three.

According to John Cairns, a professor at Harvard University School of Public Health: 'The majority of cancers cannot be cured by radiation, because the dose of X-rays required to kill all the cancer cells would also kill the patient.' (*Scientific American*, November 1985) This contrasts markedly with the views of the US National Cancer Institute quote at the beginning of this chapter: 'Radiation therapy is an effective way to treat many kinds of cancer in almost any part of the body.'

I know who I believe.

Chemotherapy

According to the National Cancer Institute, chemotherapy drugs can produce cures in about fifteen per cent of cancer cases. According to less enthusiastic experts, the figure is really five per cent: 'In some cancers, chemotherapy can cause the tumors to disappear. In other cases, chemotherapy makes the tumor shrink [or] may at least stop the tumor from growing or make it grow more slowly. There are some cases, however, in which chemotherapy has no effect on the growth of the tumor.' (Morra and Potts, 1980)

The writers, strong proponents of conventional cancer treatment, go on to warn their readers that chemotherapy needs to be administered by specialists trained in its use: 'Patients who are not closely monitored could die from the side-effects, because the drugs are very potent.' The situation has not changed since these comments were made. There has been no chemotherapeutic revolution.

What does chemotherapy involve?
Chemotherapy simply means that chemical substances are used to treat a medical problem. Taking aspirin for a headache is a relatively innocuous form of chemotherapy (though 750 people a year die in the US from aspirin abuse!). As applied to cancer treatment, chemotherapy involves the use of very powerful chemical substances. Over one hundred different drugs can be used, either alone or in combination. These drugs are poisonous. They kill normal cells in the same way they kill cancer cells because, to date, it has not been possible to develop a cancer-specific chemotherapeutic agent.

Chemotherapy drugs act generally by killing DNA or the DNA synthesising process. Those that simply attack the DNA will affect normal cells just as much as the cancer

77

cells. Those that focus on the synthesising process will attack all fast-dividing cells – including the cells that line the intestinal tract, blood-forming and hair cells. Anyone taking one of these agents will suffer some degree of nausea and perhaps infection. These infections can be life threatening. It is not uncommon for people undergoing chemotherapy to develop pneumonia for example – some dying as a result.

A random sampling of the side-effects someone taking chemotherapy can expect to suffer are: mouth sores, bone marrow suppression, liver and/or kidney damage, skin darkening, nail damage, fluid retention, high blood pressure, heart damage, bleeding internally and externally and lowered blood calcium. Some of these are more general than others. Liver and kidney damage, along with bone marrow suppression, are the most widespread. Different agents have different effects.* In addition, some, if not the majority, of chemotherapeutic agents are themselves carcinogenic – i.e. they will cause cancer in a number of cases.

If anyone should doubt the reality of the seriousness of the side-effects, let them consider this. According to Dr Gerald Dermer, author of *The Immortal Cell*, in some drug trials as many as twenty per cent of cancer patients died not from the disease but from the chemotherapy – so-called 'toxic deaths'. These trials are done on people with advanced cancers who are therefore recommended by doctors for clinical trials.

There appear to be a large number of toxic deaths associated with high-dose chemotherapy treatments. The more intractable cancers appear to be, and the more desperate researchers are to show some effect, the more likely they are to use high-dose treatment regimes. This does not benefit patients. Often the dose given is so lethal that it kills the bone marrow. This requires that patients undergo a procedure known as autologous bone marrow transplantation, in which some of their bone marrow is taken out before the chemotherapy treatments and cultivated. At the end of the treatments, this marrow is then transplanted back into the patient. This is an expensive, high-tech and gruelling treat-

---

* Anyone taking adriamycin or any of its variations (doxorubicin, epirubicin, etc.), for example, is advised to take co-enzyme Q-10 before, during and after treatment to protect the heart.

ment, which appears to have some short-term benefit in increasing disease free periods, but no long-term benefits in terms of increased survival.

Former US Vice-President Hubert Humphrey, who died from bladder cancer, called chemotherapy 'bottled death'. As with radiation, side-effects are to be expected from chemotherapy because damage to the body is inevitable. One study reported that from 1965 to 1969, the one-year survival rate for colon cancer was sixty-eight per cent, but that this fell to sixty-five per cent over the next two years, 1970–71. The reason was that it was being treated more vigorously with chemotherapy.

The successes of chemotherapy

However, some cancers have shown a very positive response to chemotherapy. It has been shown to be very effective in the treatment of: Burkitt's lymphoma, Hodgkin's disease, non-Hodgkin's lymphoma, acute lymphocytic leukaemia, choriocarcinoma, embryonal testicular cancer, Ewing's sarcoma, lymphosarcoma, retinoblastoma, rhabdomyosarcoma and Wilms' tumour. Unfortunately, together, these account for only five per cent of all cancer cases.

The success rate in these cancers varies. The best responders are the lymphomas and the leukaemias. In the case of non-Hodgkin's lymphoma, low-grade (slow-growing) tumours are incurable by any regime, but medium- and high-grade tumours have a good response to chemotherapy, with cure rates estimated at fifty to eighty per cent.

The most common form of leukaemia in children is the kind that responds best to chemotherapy. When leukaemia affects adults, it tends to be a less responsive form – though a five-year survival rate of fifty per cent is still claimed. Unfortunately, chemotherapy will almost certainly cause serious side-effects to children. Toxicity effects have been described as 'horrendous' – in one study sixty-one per cent suffered seizures. Strokes and other 'acute mental status changes' are high frequency effects. It also causes immune system collapse and children often have to spend months at a time in germ-free zones. However, these effects may seem inconsequential compared with the riches of life thus saved.

In one Australian case, parents of a girl with leukaemia

79

felt otherwise. On the diagnosis, they decided to give themselves six weeks to experiment with megadoses of vitamin C. They gave her 20 gm a day and six weeks later her blood counts were back to normal. Anecdotal? Undoubtedly. But nevertheless, for me, it is persuasive. Leukaemia has a number of symptoms identical to scurvy, so the vitamin C option should not be discounted out of hand.

The failures of chemotherapy
Even such a cancer research establishment figure as Harvard Medical School's Geoffrey Cooper has admitted the poor prognosis for the chemotherapy treatment of most cancers: 'Unfortunately, curative chemotherapy for most common adult malignancies (e.g. breast, colon and lung carcinomas) remains elusive,' he says in *The Cancer Book*. 'Chemotherapy of metastatic disease usually fails. Advances in chemotherapy have led to successes against a few malignancies, but not against the majority of common cancers.'

Nevertheless, chemotherapy remains a form of treatment commonly prescribed for all sorts of cancers. In many cases, doctors will point to its evident effects on chemical markers indicating the presence of cancer. But these effects are almost always temporary. This must be a very frustrating experience for oncologists, but it is certainly no reason for them to persevere in this futile exercise – yet persevere they do.

Patients are rarely told that there is a high incidence of leukaemia associated with a number of common chemotherapy drugs – up to seventeen per cent of patients over four years, according to Dr DeVita, author of cancer textbook *Cancer, Principles and Practice of Oncology*. In addition, some studies have shown that chemotherapy often accelerates the speed at which a cancer progresses after a relapse occurs. Doctors may talk encouragingly of a sixty per cent response rate, but patients need to understand that there is no connection between 'response rates' and long-term survival.

Why is chemotherapy still so commonly used?
The simple fact is, chemotherapy is big business: in 1989, it was worth US $2,400 million to the pharmaceutical companies.

80

To give some idea of the extent of those resources, every year more than 50,000 materials are tested. In fact, the major proportion of the money donated to cancer research goes to the search for chemotherapeutic drugs. It's a lucrative business for the institutes engaged in cancer research, and also for private oncologists. There have been accusations that patients have been put on ineffective low doses for long periods of time just to ensure they keep coming back. No-one wants to kill the goose that lays the golden egg. This may seem like a cheap and unsupported accusation against respectable, hard-working doctors. Yet some doctors have stated publicly that it is better for patients to be kept on a useless regime of chemotherapy rather than allow them to explore the unorthodox avenues.

Dr Charles Moertel, of the prestigious Mayo Clinic, investigated the value of one of the most common of chemotherapy agents, 5-FU, in combination with other chemotherapy agents. He found that only about fifteen to twenty per cent of patients with gastro-intestinal cancers had any form of response, and that for most of them these responses were partial and transient: 'There is no solid evidence that treatment with [5-FU and related compounds] contributes to the overall survival of patients with gastro-intestinal cancer, regardless of the stage of the disease at which they are applied.' (Moertel, 1978, quoted by Pauling, 1986)

Moertel also, according to Pauling, came to the same conclusion with regard to the effect of 5-FU in combination with other chemotherapeutic agents for a variety of cancers, from the throat to the rectum. It would seem to follow that 5-FU and related chemotherapeutic agents were contra-indicated for these cancers. But Moertel goes on to say: 'By no means, however, should these conclusions imply that these efforts should be abandoned. Patients with advanced gastro-intestinal cancer and their families have a compelling need for a basis of hope. If such hope is not offered, they will quickly seek it from the hands of quacks and charlatans.'

Moertel was writing in 1978. In 1994, *Everyone's Guide to Cancer Therapy*, the official version of orthodox cancer medicine as seen fit for the lay public, mentions the use of 5-FU with the following cancers: anal, bile-duct, bladder, breast, cervical, colorectal, oesophageal, gall-bladder, gastro-intestinal tract, head and neck, liver, ovarian, pancreatic, penile, small intestine, stomach, uterine, vaginal and vulva. To be fair, it doesn't always recommend its use. For example, in the case of bile-duct cancer it says: 'Studies have not shown that chemotherapy can prolong survival, but the standard drugs used (mitomycin-C or 5-fluorouracil) may cause tumors to shrink and help about twenty-five per cent of patients. However, patients may not be better off after chemotherapy. The treatment has side-effects and the tumor ultimately re-grows.' (Dollinger *et al*, 1994)

Therefore, in the opinion of the best informed doctors, 5-FU doesn't work – and yet it is still sufficiently commonly used to be called a 'standard drug' for the treatment of a number of cancers. New claims are now being made for the combination of 5-FU with levamisole for a number of cancers – there are claims of a thirty per cent reduction in tumour recurrence over five years for colon cancer, for example. But, as we have seen earlier, five-year survival rates cannot be trusted.

The message seems to be: it hasn't worked, so we must try harder to make it work. It is extremely worrying that the medical profession seems so wedded to chemotherapy that they would rather use a useless chemotherapeutic agent – or convince themselves of its value – than contemplate alternative therapies.

Why doesn't chemotherapy work?
The main problem is resistance. Chemotherapy is often quite successful at first. After its use, the tumour shrinks and the chemical markers in the blood decline. These markers are indications of the cancer's presence and its degree of activity. But then, even though the drugs are still being given, there is a relapse and the cancer starts to grow again. Resistance is not only common – it is the norm. This has led doctors to use two or more chemotherapy agents in combination. Yet once resistance to one drug combination occurs, there is an increased likelihood that there will be resistance to other combinations.

Cancer cells resist chemotherapy by a process known as gene amplification. This is what cancer cells do anyway – so chemotherapeutic drugs are making the cells more cancer-ous. The more they are attacked, the stronger they get. In addition, some chemotherapy drugs, known as alkylating agents, are recognised by the experts as causing bladder cancer and leukaemia. In 1985, a prominent cancer researcher, Robert T. Schimke, publicly announced the problem in a lecture at the National Institutes of Health, when he explained that cancer cells resist chemotherapy, and that resistance mimics the very processes of cancer itself.

Why are doctors still using chemotherapy?

This is a good question. It is clear that chemotherapy is a paradigm that is very attractive to anyone engaged in cancer treatment. Give the patient a drug and make the disease go away. The more powerful the drug the better. Powerful drugs enhance the doctor's status.

That is not the only reason, however. Critics of chemo-therapy have alleged far more damning reasons for the continuing use of toxic chemical agents. One, Dr Alan S. Levin, accused the pharmaceutical industry of manipulating special interests into coercing doctors to use chemothera-peutic drugs. One way is through medical insurance. In California, doctors who use 5-FU to treat colon cancer will be reimbursed, even though it is widely accepted that 5-FU doesn't work. If they use high doses of vitamin C, they will not be reimbursed. Instead, they will be in great danger of losing their medical licences.

Levin also accuses the drug companies of manipulating their experimental results. According to Dr Levin, any patient who dies during a drug trial is eliminated from the results. So, too, in many cases, are groups of patients who do not show good responses. By concentrating only on the group who respond well and eliminating the others, the drug will appear to be more effective than it really is. Even then, the final results very rarely show more than a few per cent improvement in life expectancy or tumour-free sur-vival.

So, who is this crank who suggests that pharmaceutical companies doctor their clinical trial results and coerce doctors into performing medically useless and highly dan-gerous treatments? At the time of these remarks, Dr Levin was Adjunct Associate Professor of Immunology and Dermatology at the University of California, San Francisco, School of Medicine – no 'quack'.

On examining this evidence, I can come to no other conclusion than that chemotherapy is a dangerous and desperate approach to the treatment of any cancer, except for the treatment of a few childhood and lymphatic cancers where its benefits have been well established.

Sadly, the oncologist, who recommends chemotherapy as a precaution perhaps, in talking privately face to face with the patient, will always carry a lot of weight. But do oncologists with cancer themselves opt for chemotherapy? Not necessarily. In 1986, McGill Cancer Center scientists sent a questionnaire to 118 doctors – who routinely recommended patients for clinical trials involving chemotherapeutic agents – at Princess Margaret Hospital in Toronto. The doctors were asked, if they had cancer, which of six chemotherapy treatment plans would they choose for themselves. Only seventy-nine replied, and of these, fifty-eight said they would not consent to enter any chemotherapy trial. The reasons? The ineffectiveness of chemotherapy and the unacceptably high degree of toxicity . . . This result has been supported by informal polls elsewhere.

Other standard treatments

Biological therapies

Everyone accepts that the body has an immune system
which helps to defend it against disease. This system is
generally seen at the level of specialised blood cells, called
macrophages, which recognise an invading foreign threat to
the system – i.e. a bacterium or virus. They engulf these
antigens and break them down to smaller proteins. Macrophages also release substances called cytokines, which alert
other cells, the lymphocytes, to respond. There are two
types of lymphocyte: B lymphocytes, which produce antibodies, and T lymphocytes, which have the task of record-
ing and memorising the antigens for the future. They also
attack foreign invaders directly. There are other cells such as
the white blood cells, whose job is to eat up the foreign
invaders and destroy them.

The idea behind biological therapies is that these defences
can be activated to target cancer cells – and if they can be
activated, the cancer cell will be destroyed by the body's own
immune system. Sometimes this happens spontaneously. In
1986, Molly O'Connor, a five-month-old baby, was diagnosed with neural blastoma, which had already spread to the
liver. The cancer tumour swelled up and distended the
stomach. The specialists, however, detected certain signs that
were positive and decided not to proceed with chemotherapy.
Instead, they observed her. At a certain point, the cancer
stopped growing and retreated of its own accord. She is still
alive to this day. This was a case of spontaneous remission.
Somehow the immune system kicked in, and once it had
done so, the cancer tumour disappeared.

In order to replicate this process, a large number of biological substances, extracted from tumour and immune cells, have
been investigated: interleukins, interferons, tumour necrosis

factor, prostaglandin and others. All of these substances have been trialled on cancer patients. Some have very minor side-effects, some cause flu-like symptoms and some, such as interleukin-2, have severe and life-threatening effects

This is a relatively new form of treatment, still highly experimental in its strategies and substances used. There is no doubt that some previously terminal patients are alive today because of this form of treatment.

Vaccination is another form of biological therapy. One pioneer in this field is Dr Donald Morton, Director of the John Wayne Cancer Institute. He has used the standard BCG vaccination with some success against malignant melanoma – four of the first seven patients to receive the BCG survived. That is to say, the results were magnificent – fifty per cent effectiveness in otherwise fatal conditions – but did not amount to a one hundred per cent effective cure for cancer. Analysis of the results showed that those patients whose melanoma was confined to the skin recovered, but those whose melanoma had struck deep into the body – particularly the brain – did not.

Another leading US research centre is at Johns Hopkins Hospital in Baltimore. There they have found that cervical cancer in mice responds well to vaccines – mainly because of its viral origins. Human trials are the next step. German investigators are working with vaccines based on a group of proteins called peptides, with some success. Two patients, both with advanced cancers and working with researchers in Frankfurt, were injected with vaccines containing their own cancer cells, and are now symptom free.

A vaccine against cancer? This is good news, and spells great hope for the future. Vaccination has many benefits over chemotherapy – it is potentially effective and it is non-toxic. There is even the good news that cancers of the breast, lung and prostate also responded to the melanoma-specific vaccine. If mainstream medicine is likely to come up with any cancer cure, this seems the most likely route. It is a product of scientific medicine of the right kind. But it is still early days – many research hoops have to be gone through.

Bone marrow transplantation
There are two grounds on which a patient may be advised to undergo bone marrow transplantation. One is allogenic

transplantation, in which new bone marrow – usually from a close relative without cancer – is transplanted into the patient to help the body to fight the cancer. Identical twins are fortunate in having a walking supply of perfect bone marrow to draw on. Autologous transplantation is used when the doctors want to use massive doses of chemotherapy – dose levels that would normally kill the bone marrow cells. In this case, the bone marrow is taken out before the chemotherapy course and replaced afterwards. This is perhaps the most dangerous and painful procedure known to modern medicine. The risks of death from the procedure alone are very high. It claims a success rate of forty to sixty per cent in the case of early stage leukaemias and some lymphomas – declining to ten per cent with late-stage cancers. Often it is a time-buying exercise. Apart from a few cancers such as testicular cancer and possibly breast cancer, solid tumours do not generally respond well to this procedure.

Hormones
Hormone treatment is often recommended with breast and prostate cancers. Hormonal intervention with these two cancers, however, is very different.

FOR BREAST CANCER
It has long been known that a majority of breast cancers respond to hormones. For this reason, the removal of the ovaries was a common treatment. This has been superseded by hormonal drugs, such as tamoxifen, which is taken orally, and has few side-effects. It should be taken for at least five years, though doctors may suggest that two years is adequate. About half of patients with hormone-responsive breast tumours will get good results.

FOR PROSTATE CANCER
Hormones cannot cure prostate cancer, but they can slow the growth. The idea behind the treatment is that the male hormone, testosterone, helps prostate cancer cells to thrive. Removing this hormone slows the rate of growth. One way in which this can be done is through surgical castration. Another way is through oral hormone pills that feminise the patient. The side-effects of this therapy are often severe –

besides breast development and body hair loss, there can be deep-vein thrombosis (blood clotting). In fact, the side-effects of all such drugs should be considered with care. Those for hydrocortisone, one of the drugs used, include raised blood pressure, heart trouble, mood changes, blood clots, thinning of the bone leading to increases in fractures, bruising, changes in vision and acne. It doesn't include loss of sexual interest, though this too will almost certainly happen.

Sometimes the chest may be irradiated to stop the oestrogen causing breast formation – the result can be painful. The difficulty is that these hormones have to be taken for life. Taking hormones for prostate cancer is clearly a tough option – very severe side-effects have to be borne, for a less than satisfactory objective.

Hyperthermia

This refers to the raising of the temperature of the body to about 108° F (42° C), or higher, by various means. The whole body may be heated, or localised heating can be achieved using microwaves. There is some disagreement as to its usefulness. At present, heating treatments are generally limited to one-hour sessions, but it appears that longer sessions have achieved some exciting results – the longer the better. This is, in fact, a therapy that has crossed the orthodox-alternative divide and is recommended by both.

Since the high heat interferes with the cell's ability to repair itself after radiation treatments, heat treatment is now being used along with radiation, and it appears that immediate response rates nearly double as a result. One study showed that radiation on its own had a thirty-one to thirty-seven per cent response rate, while radiation with heat treatment had a response rate of sixty-three to seventy-one per cent. This suggests that if radiation is to be chosen as the form of treatment, the best way of conducting it may be to have very small fractions of daily radiation, with long-term hyperthermia treatment in-between.

Laser treatments

This involves focusing a beam of high-intensity light at tumour cells. Its use is restricted at present to treating pre-cancerous states and small tumours. It works by vaporising tissue at very high temperatures. The result of laser

88

treatment can be a hole, or an ulcer. This treatment, however, can only be used against the portion of a tumour showing on the surface – but tumours are like icebergs. For cervical pre-cancerous conditions, it is claimed to be very effective – for all other purposes it hasn't definitely been demonstrated that it is curative.

Common cancers – the standard orthodox treatments

Bladder cancer
One of the top ten cancers in terms of incidence. It occurs three to four times more frequently in men than women and the main cause is smoking. It generally strikes late in life. Blood in the urine is the most common symptom.

Surgery: Most common. This involves removal of the bladder. As one expert puts it, this removal: 'will bring about quite a major change in your life style and it is important that you are prepared as well as possible for it'. A radical operation will affect the patient's sex life. Five-year survival – fifty to ninety per cent, depending on age.

Radiotherapy: Used sometimes as an alternative to surgery, but the results are not so good.

Chemotherapy: No demonstrable impact from the use of chemotherapy.

Brain cancer
Approximately 4,000 cases a year in the UK. Two groups most affected: children and the middle-aged.

Surgery: The main treatment, with the aim of removing as much tumour tissue as possible.

Radiation: Does not have much effect.

Chemotherapy: Increasingly used to treat brain cancers in children, though without much success. In the words of one oncologist: 'The chemotherapy of brain tumours has consistently been among the most disappointing failures in clinical oncology, achieving at best only a short-term palliation.' Five-year survival is nearly sixty per cent for children and twenty-six per cent for those under forty-five.

Breast cancer

Every year, 30,000 women in Britain are diagnosed with breast cancer. Professor Michael Braun suggests that, even without any form of treatment, probably thirty per cent of such cancers will not proceed, but will be self-limiting – i.e. even without treatment, they will not pose a threat to the patient's health. High tendency to spread.

Surgery: Lumpectomy with radiation has as good results as mastectomy. In Austria, some success is being achieved with the injection of Wobe Mugos enzymes along with lumpectomy (without radiation).

Radiation: Lumpectomy with radiation appears to have better results than without radiation, but there are the risks associated with radiation. Doctors downplay risks, but no figures are available.

Chemotherapy: Up to 1994, 230 trials round the world on chemotherapy for advanced breast cancer have been conducted. None provide evidence that survival is prolonged. More aggressive chemotherapy regimes are associated with reduced survival rates. Survival rates in the 1950s seem to have been better than survival rates after the introduction of chemotherapy. Recent reports of a five per cent improvement in survivability since the introduction of chemotherapy as a standard post-operative therapy appear to be correct – but no-one is sure whether this is due to chemotherapy or some other cause.

Critics say treatment of breast cancer has gone from too much surgery to too much chemotherapy, with little impact on survival. One interesting idea being tried out in some hospitals is to use chemotherapy before surgery – this takes advantage of the short-term shrinking effect to reduce the size of the tumour being cut out. The benefits of this approach will not be known for some time.

Hormone treatment: One interesting early success with breast cancer was to reduce the amount of hormones around the cancer by chemical means, but this is not much done nowadays. Hormone treatment with tamoxifen seems to be associated with slight benefits. Unfortunately, it has been associated with uterine cancer of the endometrium.

Cancer of unknown primary site (CUPS)

This is first detected when a secondary metastasis is found, but the primary tumour cannot be identified. This may be because the primary site is small or in a location that is difficult to detect. About 5,000 cases in the UK annually. Prognosis is generally poor, though some such cancers can be cured if the primary can be located and if it is found to be a cancer with a good cure rate by orthodox means.

Given the prognosis if the primary is not found, there are no standard treatments, though chemotherapy is often offered. Individual metastases may be surgically removed and the area irradiated – but the chances that orthodox treatment of any metastatic cancer will be successful are not good. Radiotherapy may be used if the primary is thought likely to be in the head/neck area. The impact of any such attempt is likely to be damaging, and aggressive treatment of secondaries will probably not be beneficial in the long term.

Cervical and uterine cancer

In Britain, 9,000 women a year are affected. Most cancers in this area are slow growing, but about one per cent are very aggressive.

Surgery: Hysterectomy is generally advised. This has a thirty per cent complication rate.

Radiation: If surgery is not an option, then radiation is the only orthodox treatment available. The risk of damage is very high, given the number of organs in this area. Almost certainly the upper vagina will atrophy or be scarred, making sexual relations difficult or impossible. It will bring on the menopause.

Chemotherapy: No significant survival advantage has been reported for the use of radiation and chemotherapy combined. An immediate response rate has been shown, but the tumour almost always returns.

Colon cancer

About six per cent of all cancers in the UK are in the colon. Around 20,000 men and women are affected – and another 12,000 have cancer of the rectum. High fibre diets help to protect against these cancers.

Surgery: For colon cancer, half the colon is typically

removed. For the rectum, radiation to reduce the size of the tumour prior to surgery allows the sphincter muscle to be retained in eighty-five per cent of cases. If the tumour is low down, this is not possible, and the entire rectum is removed. There is a high incidence of impotence and problems in the urinary system (estimated twenty-five to forty per cent).

Radiation: Has not proved to extend survival.

Chemotherapy: In some studies, treatment with 5-FU and levamisole has shown a thirty per cent improvement in three-year survival rates for Grade 3 colon cancers – but not for Grade 2 or Grade 4. Levamisole is extremely toxic, and considered to be a long-term poison. Given alone, it substantially decreases survival by about half. Early supporters of 5-FU and levamisole are back-tracking. No other chemotherapy regime works. There has been no improvement in overall survivability of colon cancer cases.

Kaposi's sarcoma

An otherwise rare cancer, it is an almost inevitable consequence of AIDS. This disease causes lesions in a wide variety of places, internally and externally. Lesions on the lung have a poor prognosis, while those in the digestive tract cause little problem. It is not considered curable, but it can be managed.

Radiation: The lesions are sensitive to small doses of radiation, which are not too uncomfortable.

Chemotherapy: The problem with using standard chemotherapy, even if it were shown to work, is that it would almost certainly depress the immune system, hardly beneficial for someone with AIDS or HIV. However, highly dilute injections of chemotherapeutic agents into each specific lesion appear to have some benefits without depressing overall immune levels.

Biological therapy: Agents such as alpha-interferon have had some success.

Kidney and ureter

Smoking is a high risk factor. In the UK, about 4,400 new patients are diagnosed annually. Five-year survival is twenty to sixty per cent, depending on age and sex; elderly women patients fare worst.

Surgery: Removal of the affected kidneys and possibly surrounding tissue.

Radiation: No benefits have been demonstrated.

Chemotherapy: There may be, at best, a five to ten per cent effect in producing a complete regression.

Biological therapy: Interferon alpha reduces tumours in ten to thirty per cent of patients. Interleukin-2, with patients' own LAK or TIL cells, has had some success.

Leukaemia

There are four main types of leukaemia – two are acute and progress rapidly, while two others are chronic, developing slowly. All are cancers of the white cells in the bone marrow or the lymph nodes. Chronic leukaemias tend to affect the middle-aged and older. Taken together, there are approximately 7,000 new cases a year in Britain.

TYPE 1: CHRONIC LYMPHOCYTIC LEUKAEMIA (CLL)

Steroids/chemotherapy: Often left untreated at first, but later these two treatments may be used. Cure is unlikely, but can be controlled by medication for periods of time.

TYPE 2: CHRONIC MYELOGENOUS LEUKAEMIA (CML)

Chemotherapy: First line of attack, followed by bone marrow transplantation from a member of the family. Twenty per cent of patients undergoing this procedure die as a direct result of the operation. However, this is the only standard treatment that offers a chance of a cure.

TYPE 3: ACUTE LYMPHOBLASTIC LEUKAEMIA (ALL)

Chemotherapy: This is the leukaemia that attacks the young. Children have a good chance of recovery with chemotherapy – but there are serious side-effects that need to be put into the equation. This leukaemia has the best prognosis, with five-year survival rate of thirty to seventy-three per cent, depending on age.

TYPE 4: ACUTE MYELOBLASTIC LEUKAEMIA (AML)

Chemotherapy/ bone marrow transplantation: Intensive treatment can achieve three-year survival of twenty per cent of patients with this condition.

Liver cancer

Symptoms – abdominal pains, fevers, nausea – are often missed. There are only 1,500 cases a year in the UK.

Surgery: If the tumour is restricted to one of the liver's two lobes it can be removed – if not, surgery is not advised unless for a liver transplant.

Radiation: Sometimes used after surgery – but not advised, as it is very damaging to normal liver cells.

Chemotherapy: No evidence that chemotherapy has any beneficial effect.

Cryosurgery: The cancer cells are frozen. No information is available as to efficacy.

Lung cancer – small cell

Twenty to twenty-five per cent of all lung cancer cases. Also known as oat cell carcinoma of the lung. Less than ten per cent of patients obtain long-term remission. In UK, there are 45,000 new lung cancer cases a year in total.

Surgery: No benefit.

Radiation: Heavy radiation doses are required to the chest and occasionally to the brain, because of frequent metastases there. Radiation of the brain does not prolong survival.

Chemotherapy: This has a proven effect on survivability – people taking chemotherapy live for a few weeks or months longer on average, although not years. There is disagreement over whether radiation alone or in combination with chemotherapy shows the greater life-enhancing benefits. Some patients die from the treatment.

Lung cancer – non-small cell

Seventy-five to eighty per cent of lung cancers are of this kind. Five-year survival is eight to ten per cent.

Surgery: This is the mainstay of treatment.

Radiation: This may be done instead of surgery.

Chemotherapy: No study has shown chemotherapy to be more than marginally beneficial – and the regimes used are highly toxic.

Lymphomas – Hodgkin's disease
Only about 1,500 cases a year in the UK.
Radiation/chemotherapy: Seventy to eighty per cent can be cured with these treatments.

Lymphomas – non-Hodgkin's
7,000 cases a year in the UK. Low-grade lymphomas are considered incurable, but average survivability is six to twelve years. Not normally an aggressive cancer, it can take an aggressive form.
Chemotherapy: Although the lumps respond readily, they usually return. High-grade lymphomas are forty to fifty per cent curable, and best treated with chemotherapy.
Radiotherapy: Very early stage lymphomas may have prolonged responses to radiation.

Malignant melanoma
Accounts for one to two per cent of cancer deaths. Five-year survival is better for women (seventy-five per cent) than men (fifty-two per cent). There are fewer than 5,000 cases in the UK each year.
Surgery: Surgical removal of tumour is generally done.
Radiation: Melanoma cells are resistant to radiation, but it can be recommended to shrink a node.
Chemotherapy: No proven long-term benefits from standard chemotherapy, although temporary responses can be achieved.
Other: Vaccination with BCG and specific anti-melanoma vaccine has had good results in the US.

Oesophageal
Risk factors are: age, long-term drinking and smoking and consumption of pickled vegetables. Contributing factors are diets deficient in vitamins B2 and B3, magnesium and zinc. Higher per-capita incidence in UK than US – about 6,000 cases a year in the UK (compared with 11,000 in US). Usually diagnosed late. Prognosis is poor – five-year survival is less than ten per cent.

Surgery: Removal of tumours in lower section of oesophagus. May involve radical surgery of surrounding area. Only to be done in specialist centres, as five to ten per cent of patients do not survive radical operation.

Radiation: May cure patients with very small lesions – otherwise used only to support surgery or to help reduce symptoms.

Chemotherapy: Used mainly to shrink lesions before surgery.

Ovarian cancer

Ovarian cancer has a high incidence in most industrialised states, but extremely low in Japan. It affects approximately 6,000 women a year in the UK. The cause is unknown. Unfortunately, most women have advanced cancer when diagnosed, due to absence of early symptoms. Five-year survival rate is fifteen to forty-four per cent, depending on age.

Surgery: Removal of ovaries at early stage, or 'de-bulking' of a large tumour. De-bulking usually requires radical surgery to neighbouring organs and tissues.

Radiation: Sometimes used instead of chemotherapy.

Chemotherapy: This is standard. Good response rates (forty to eighty per cent).There is some indication that chemotherapy may extend life by a year or so, but there is no clear evidence of this.

Pancreatic cancer

In the UK, 7,000 people a year get this cancer. Five-year survival is only four per cent.

Surgery: 'Surgery is rarely curative but can be used for palliation,' says one textbook – though radical surgery, called the Whipple procedure, may be feasible if the tumour is small and no lymph nodes are involved. This procedure is not often indicated, but has a twenty-two per cent five-year survival record.

Radiation: Sometimes recommended, but carries a very high risk of damaging kidneys, spleen, liver, spinal cord and the bowel.

Chemotherapy: No evidence of positive effects from chemotherapy. Despite this, thirty per cent of patients receive chemotherapy.

Prostate cancer

Affects one per cent of men under fifty, rising to half of men over eighty. As a generally slow-growing cancer, little benefit gained from screening. Most men die without knowing they have had it. Five-year survival is forty-three per cent. It is not related to the problem of an enlarged prostate, or frequency of having sex. It appears to be an illness associated with age, with the US (where the death rate is high compared with other countries) and urban life. Approximately 14–15,000 men are diagnosed in the UK each year. PSA screening methods are of debatable value as they may be normal when cancer is present and abnormal with benign problems. PSA levels fluctuate wildly.

Surgery: Often recommended, and will cure if cancer has not spread beyond prostate. However, it leads to sexual impotence and possibly to urinary incontinence.

Radiation: The same problems as surgery (impotence, etc.), with the added possibility of being left in permanent pain.

Chemotherapy: No beneficial effect.

Hormone treatment: Severe side-effects. Does not cure, but slows growth rate.

Cryosurgery: Freezing of the prostate. Still experimental, and the side-effects versus effectiveness question has not been answered.

Other: Patients often choose to wait and see what happens, which many doctors approve of.

Sarcomas

Rare, affecting the muscle and bone tissues, and requiring very careful management. These cancers tend to affect children, teenagers and young adults – though some attack older age groups (forty to sixty). They are very aggressive, although survival has improved dramatically. One risk factor is exposure to radiation.

Surgery: If indicated, surgery is radical and often involves amputation.

Radiation: Used before and after surgery.

Chemotherapy: Children benefit more than adults – but suffer severe side-effects.

Skin cancer – non-melanoma

The most common cancer found in humans. In the UK, it comes second behind lung cancer. Incidence appears to be increasing. Half of men over sixty-five are believed to have at least one skin cancer. The cure rate is very high, with a five-year survival of around ninety-seven per cent. It affects fair skins exposed to the sun.

Curettage and electro-desiccation (C&E): This involves a sharp-tipped instrument. Bleeding is controlled by an electrical instrument. Used on small lesions with distinct boundaries. Low risk.

Cryosurgery: Liquid nitrogen is used to freeze the skin. Low risk.

Surgery: Mohs micrographic surgery is used to remove the skin in horizontal layers, to remove the lesion. This is time consuming and requires expertise – may need plastic surgery as a follow-up. Surgery may also involve use of lasers.

Radiation: This involves a low-penetration radiation beam. Radiation should not be used on patients under the age of fifty, as treatment can cause new cancers to grow at radiation site. It also makes recurrences more difficult to deal with, as radiation makes lesions more aggressive and resistant. Leaves white blemishes. Treated areas will be inflamed for four to six weeks.

Chemotherapy: 5-FU may be given as a cream, but results can be deceptive – the surface of the lesion may die, while the internal base continues. Up to fifty per cent of lesions treated in this way return.

Other: Photodynamic therapy (see page 280 for details).

Stomach cancer

Once very common, the incidence of this cancer has declined over the last fifty years – for no known reason. Around 13,000 cases a year in the UK. If caught early, fifty per cent cure rate, but otherwise prognosis is poor, with five-year survival ten to eleven per cent.

Surgery: Requires radical surgical removal of entire stomach, with surrounding lymph nodes. Up to fifteen per cent of patients do not survive the operation, and complications are common.

Radiation: Not used to cure, but may help to reduce

symptoms. May be used before operation, as a Japanese study showed this slightly improves success rate.

Chemotherapy: No benefits have been demonstrated, although about ten per cent are treated with chemotherapy.

Testicular cancer
About 1,500 cases a year in the UK. It has a very good five-year survival rate (ninety+ per cent). No known causes. A major cause of cancer among men aged between twenty and forty.

Surgery: Affected testis is removed. New techniques allow men to retain both potency and fertility.

Radiation: Common, but probably unnecessary.

Chemotherapy: Possibly unnecessary in early stage cases. Combination chemotherapy is used with good regression rates.

Further information
These brief summaries are for indication only. For those who wish to investigate more fully the standard treatments for their cancers, they should read two general books, *Everyone's Guide to Cancer Therapy* and *What You Really Need to Know about Cancer*. Please bear in mind that prognosis information is from orthodox sources, and does not necessarily apply to patients who decide to follow complementary or alternative treatments.

The Physicians' Data Query (PDQ) System is the most up-to-date cancer information system available for standard orthodox and investigational treatments anywhere in the world. There is separate information for patients and doctors – although patients are free to access the information available to doctors. The information is updated every month. It can be accessed on the Internet by anyone with a computer and modem. Look for CancerNet. One third of people using this system do so from outside the US.[4]

Reducing the side-effects of radiation and chemotherapy

Although I have been very critical of standard cancer treatments, many patients have undergone these therapies, their tumours have disappeared and they appear to be living comfortable lives. In the US, it is estimated that there are eight million people who have recovered following orthodox treatment. The therapeutic conveyor belt will continue to channel patients to these therapies in large numbers, with many patients feeling happy that their cancer is in the hands of the experts.

For these and other reasons, radiation and chemotherapy will continue to be used for the foreseeable future. However, since these forms of treatment are hazardous, anyone deciding to undergo either of them should consider the advice of a number of complementary therapists, taking the following precautions before, during and after treatment.

Aloe vera
Some people recommend drinking aloe vera juice regularly for its healing properties. We have already noted the impact of radiation on the intestines. Rub aloe vera gel into skin areas affected by radiation half an hour before exposure.

Chlorophyll
Foods rich in chlorophyll, such as green cabbage, broccoli and alfalfa, have been shown to reduce radiation damage by fifty per cent in studies on guinea pigs. Chlorophyll is very similar in its molecular composition to haemoglobin.

DMSO
DMSO, dimethyl sulphoxide, an organic sulphur compound of great therapeutic value, which should be available on prescription, has shown itself to be valuable both in alleviating

the side-effects of radiation and as an anti-cancer therapy in its own right. There is evidence that, when combined with low doses of chemotherapeutic agents, it is also highly effective against cancer.

Garlic
This contains two powerful substances: allicin oil and organic germanium. It also contains something that Russian scientists have called vitamin X, because its functions are not yet fully understood (see also page 180).

Herbs
A number of herbs are useful as protective agents: Siberian ginseng, panax ginseng and chaparral. In the case of panax ginseng, a Korean study found that a normally fatal dose of radiation would leave five per cent of mice alive in the control group, compared with 82.5 per cent in the group given the herb. Chinese herbs – especially blood strengtheners and kidney tonics – have shown great ability to support the body.

Ice-pack
Some people have suggested that keeping an ice-pack on the head during the chemotherapy sessions and for an hour or so after may prevent hair loss.

Immune system boosting drugs
Isoprinosine7 is marketed under the trade names Methisoprinol and Inosiplex. It is used for anyone with a compromised immune system – AIDS and cancer patients – as it has demonstrated a strong anti-viral activity and is valuable for restoring and strengthening the immune system. It is often used post-operatively and with radiation and chemotherapy.

Iodine
Iodine deficiency can also occur as a result of radiotherapy and some form of supplementation should be considered. It affects a large number of the body's metabolic processes. For this reason, it is recommended that seaweed products such as kelp or dulce, available at any adequate health store, should become a regular part of the diet – also green

vegetables, and egg yolks. A tincture of iodine can be made up at any chemist's shop – ask for Lugol's solution.

Iron and copper
Radiation – and even ultra-violet light – causes problems for the absorption of these two minerals. Iron supplementation is therefore recommended, with vitamin C, to aid bio-availability. This will prevent radioactive plutonium replacing it in the body's iron stores – the liver, bone marrow, etc. Optimal levels of iron in the body prevent this uptake.

Lactobacillus acidophilus
These are the friendly bacteria. L. acidophilus and L. bulgaricus have a noted effect in cleaning out the toxic wastes that result from these therapies. As a result, this impact of the treatments is reduced. Start taking before any treatment is started.[5]

Magnesium
Magnesium deficiency can be caused by drinking too much milk, coffee, alcohol and fluoridated water. Deficiency can cause a loss of calcium and potassium, kidney disease, muscle cramps, irritability, depression and even heart disease. It is an important mineral, which needs to be taken as a supplement unless your diet also includes a lot of sea vegetables, soybean products or nuts.

Olive oil
When it constitutes fifteen per cent of total daily calories, olive oil provides optimal protection against radiation. In one study with mice which received from zero to thirty per cent of their diet in the form of olive oil, those mice that had no olive oil all suffered radiation damage to liver, kidneys, lungs, skin and hair. Olive oil demonstrated strong protective properties.

Potassium
Radiation causes problems for the sodium-potassium balance of the body. Potassium is a very important mineral, essential for nerves, muscles, regulation of osmotic pressure, maintenance of the acid-base balance of the body and for the proper levels of blood sugar. Ocean fish, seaweeds (kelp,

103

dulce, etc.), beans, whole grains and dried bananas are good sources. The daily requirement is 5–6,000 mg. It is best to take it in natural rather than supplement form.

Reishi mushrooms
In Japan, drinking tea made with reishi mushrooms (ling zhi) is also often recommended for radiation patients, as it protects the white blood cells.

Seaweed
Lots of sea vegetables are recommended. Anecdotal evidence strongly suggests that side-effects are much reduced if the patient takes large quantities of seaweed during treatment.

Selenium
This has a protective effect against mercury – as in dental fillings. It also helps protect against radioactivity. The daily requirement is 100–200 mg.

Silica
One side-effect of radiation is the weakening of bones. This would normally indicate calcium supplementation, but calcium is potentially dangerous for cancer patients. However, silica is converted to calcium in the body – and is in any case a superior way of taking in bio-available calcium. Some nutritionists advise that there is little proof that calcium supplementation is of any value. Lots of green leafy vegetables – organic if possible – very lightly cooked, raw or juiced will provide good quantities of calcium and silica. It is one of life's ironies that vegetarians take in more calcium than meat eaters.

Slippery elm
Since damage to the mucous membranes lining all the hollow tubes in the body is inevitable, some complementary therapists recommend that radiation patients should drink lots of slippery elm, a herbal compound that should be available at your local health shop. It is intended to replace the natural mucous material lining the insides of hollow organs. Blackcurrant juice is also recommended (and see Olive oil, above).

SOD (Superoxide Dismutase)

Fibrosis is a major debilitating side-effect of radiation treatment. The only substance known to have any beneficial impact on fibroids is SOD. It has become increasingly available at specialist health product stores.[6]

> French scientists have also shown that injections with a form of SOD called Lipsod® can be successfully used to treat long established fibrosis caused by radiation therapy. After just three weeks of intramuscular injection, fibrosis was reduced on average by one-third and significant softening occurred in eighty-two per cent of the cases. It did not matter how old the fibrosis was at the time of SOD treatment. (Moss, 1992)

SOD is also used to pre-treat patients who subsequently receive treatment with tumour necrosis factor (TNF). TNF is toxic, but the toxicity is substantially reduced by SOD injections. SOD, as with other enzymes, is apparently best injected, as stomach enzymes can easily damage it. SOD also prevented fibrosis from developing in people undergoing radiation therapy.

Sodium alginate

Sodium alginate is also highly recommended, as it helps reduce the impact of radiotherapy on the bones and, in small doses, is known to act as a cancer preventative. Brown sea vegetables, such as kelp, are a good source of sodium alginate.

Visualisation

Anyone opting for radiation and chemotherapy should develop a positive attitude to these treatments and visualise how they are working against the cancer. One experiment has shown that people with negative attitudes to these treatments do not do well, while those who are positive do much better.

Vitamin A

Both radiation and chemotherapy attack the epithelial cells that line the inside of the intestines and which produce the mucous membrane. Vitamin A is necessary for the growth and maintenance of epithelial tissue, and it is therefore

105

necessary to take it, either as vitamin A or as beta-carotene, in large quantities while undergoing either treatment. Several glasses of fresh carrot juice a day throughout the treatment would be sufficient.

Vitamin C

Previously, chemotherapy patients were urged not to take any anti-oxidant vitamins, particularly vitamin C, during their treatment, as it was believed these would reduce the treatment's effect. However, the view is now that supporting the system with vitamins may not be a bad thing.

Vitamin E

This helps the body to recover from post-irradiation anaemia and helps to protect red and white blood cells. It has been found to protect the heart against damage; lower skin toxicity from the doxorubicin agents (a family of chemicals used in chemotherapy); and protect against lung fibrosis from use of bleomycin. Taking 1,600 iu or more, starting one week before chemotherapy, has a significant impact on hair retention.

Yeast

There is good yeast – and bad yeast. One good yeast is Saccharomyces cerevisiae. A bad yeast is Candida albicans. Nutritional yeast bonds with pollutants and heavy metals. Mixed with brown rice, this has protective value for the liver. Bio-Strath is a fermented Swiss product that contains this good yeast together with fifteen herbs and other ingredients. These are added one at a time: malt extract, unrefined honey, unprocessed orange juice, and the following herbs: angelica, balm, basil, camomile, cinnamon, caraway, elder, fennel, horseradish, hyssop, lavender, licorice, peppermint, parsley, sage and thyme.

In one study, a group of radiation patients who took Bio-Strath suffered no weight loss, or depression of the haemoglobin. It also helped to enhance the assimilation of nutrients. It also has been shown to retard tumour growth in mice – and mice on a diet of Bio-Strath did not develop as many cancers as a control group.

For further information on reducing the effects of radiotherapy and chemotherapy, see *Fighting Radiation and Chemical Pollutants*, by Steven Schechter.

Cancer research

Underlying all orthodox cancer treatment is the belief that it is scientific. Both patients and doctors base their faith in modern medicine on the credo that behind everything doctors do there is a vast machinery of scientific expertise that is creating, testing and evaluating products and processes. For cancer, this system is going all out to find a cure, with no other considerations being taken into account.

Yet even a casual look at modern medicine will find little that is based on such scientific procedures. Dr Luisa Dillner, an assistant editor of the *British Medical Journal*, explains: 'Less than half of what doctors do now is based on solid scientific evidence. This is not to say that doctors are lazy or incompetent. It is partly that medicine moves so fast it is hard to keep up with the latest evidence of what works and what does not.' (*Guardian*, October 1995)

The simple fact is, there is no proof that surgery and radiation are effective methods of treatment of cancer. Chemotherapy, on the other hand, has been very heavily tested by scientific methods of extreme rigor – and found, on the whole, not to be effective.

Doctors would claim that it would be unethical to require surgery and radiation to be put to rigorous tests, because it is generally accepted within the profession that they do work. The basis of any test is doubt. If you really don't know whether a form of treatment is effective, then it is proper to do a test. If there is no doubt, then doing a test would only deprive a number of patients of treatment that would be beneficial for them, which would be unethical.

This is a good argument, as far as it goes. It may even be valid in any individual case. But medical statisticians, as we have seen, have not found much support for this position.

Dr Hardin Jones presented a paper nearly thirty years ago arguing that his overall statistical analysis suggested that no treatment was better than any treatment – indeed it was four times better! People who received no treatment were likely to live four times longer than those who did not. There has been no marked change since then.

Doctors and statisticians may be looking at different things. Since doctors focus on the disease, not the patient, they may be able to claim successful treatment, even though a patient's survivability may not be affected: the treatment was a success, even though the patient died.

'Proof' and the clinical trial

Proof, in a medical context, has a very specific meaning: something has been demonstrated to be true, in a double-blind clinical trial. This is a specialised experimental procedure, which is the end result of a series of other clinical trials. Let's look at the whole process.

The double-blind clinical trial can be applied to any practice or treatment, although most of these trials relate to the development of drugs. Usually, the initial idea is developed in the laboratory. A scientist finds a chemical agent that appears to be toxic to cancer cells in petri dishes. This is tried out on rats or mice, to see if the effect persists, and also to see what dose levels might be appropriate for humans. This is the preliminary stage. A drug is then given a phase 1 clinical trial. About twenty people – terminal patients who have volunteered – are given the drug. The sole purpose of this trial is to determine dose levels. It is not expected that any of the phase 1 patients will survive.

The next step is to see which cancer tumours are likely to be the most responsive to this new drug. Different groups of about twenty patients each, all having the same type of cancer, are tested to determine the response rate. Does the drug work better for breast or colon cancer, or what? This is the objective of the phase 2 trials, which again are conducted on patients who have no further orthodox treatment options. If the results are acceptable, then the process moves to the last phase.

The phase 3 clinical trial focuses on one particular drug regime, and applies it to thousands of patients – all with the same cancer – over a period of time. These patients are in two groups: the experimental group – which receives the new drug – and the control group, which doesn't. Instead, they get a placebo which is identical to the drug, but which contains nothing of medical benefit. It is best if the patients don't know who is receiving the drug – this is known as a blind trial. The trial becomes double-blind when even the doctors dispensing the new drug don't know who is getting it and who isn't.

In simplified terms, this is the process all new drugs go through in order to get approval for their general use. It is also the procedure used to assess the value of the drug. However, once a drug has been approved in this way, doctors will start using it in different, unapproved ways. This is admitted by the authors of *Everyone's Guide to Cancer Therapy*, who write: 'Many drug programs in standard use are not listed as "approved". They are used because experience with patients has shown they are effective.' This applies to about half of all current uses of anti-cancer drugs in the US. The critic may ask: 'Where is the science there?' The treatment is based solely on 'experience', which must first have been obtained by applying the drug randomly.

For patients recommended to join a clinical trial, the key implications of this have to be taken on board. Firstly, they should understand that apart from the clinical trial, their doctors have run out of ideas about what to do with them. Their cancer is 'terminal'. (I have put the word in inverted commas, because some patients may owe their lives to being classified as terminal, having been saved from gruelling radiation and pointless chemotherapy, and been freed to look at alternative treatments.) Secondly, patients should remember that no standard chemotherapy regimes have established themselves for the vast majority of cancers over the last twenty to thirty years. Since the clinical trials of the past two to three decades have not been successful, the chances of a new drug being successful are also remote.

It is hard to imagine that there should be any problem with the focus of modern scientific research and the means it uses to advance knowledge and thereby aid the development of cancer treatments. Unfortunately, closer examination reveals fundamental flaws.

109

FLAW ONE

Dr Gerald Dermer, who published his views in his book *The Immortal Cell*, pointed out one major flaw, so great it invalidates all laboratory-based cancer research. When most people talk about cancer they are, correctly, thinking about tumours. These tumours consist of rapidly reproducing cells, which have specific characteristics depending on what kind of cancer they are. If a breast tumour spreads to the lung, the resulting tumour is still composed of cells that have the characteristics of the original breast cancer cell. However, when cancer researchers think of cancer cells, they are thinking of the cells they observe in petri dishes in their laboratories, cells which derive from cell lines.

What are cell lines?

In 1951, a woman called 'Helen Lane' became a patient at Johns Hopkins Hospital in Baltimore, Maryland. She had cervical cancer, and eventually died of this disease – but her cells live on. Cells from her tumour were removed and placed in a petri dish, with a culture to feed them. All previous attempts to grow tumour cells outside the body had failed. 'Helen Lane's' cells successfully made the leap from existence *in vivo* (i.e. in the living body) to existence *in vitro* (i.e. in a petri dish). Forty-five years on, these cells – known as the HeLa cell line – continue to reproduce and to be used in research. 'Helen Lane's' real name was Henrietta Lacks, a black woman from Baltimore, as revealed in an article in the British *Sunday Times* in March 1997, and in a television programme. Her permission was not sought and her family, who did not know of HeLa until recently, have never benefited from her contribution to science.

It is not easy to create a cell line. Tumour cells will generally live a short time in a petri dish before dying off. But very occasionally, something else happens. One or more cells display different behaviour. They keep on dividing and do not die off. The result is a cellular culture that has evolved to living in a petri dish – it just keeps on dividing. This is the birth of an ancestral line of cells, all of which derive from this individual parent.

It is the fact that these cells grow quickly and are standardised that makes them attractive. Scientists can then conduct daily experiments on them and publish papers.

(The rule of the research game is: publish or perish.) Cell lines then provide an efficient source of cancer cells to work on. The alternative, of using fresh tumour cells, is less appealing. Malignant cells living in a tumour, just removed from a patient, are more difficult to work with. Real tumours do not just consist of malignant cancer cells – various types of normal cells are also present. Another problem is that the tumour itself remains alive for only a short period of time, so it is difficult, if not impossible, to measure the effects of experimental procedures on these living cancer cells. These difficulties slow the work, and limit the kinds of experiments that can be performed. As a result, fewer papers are published by the even fewer scientists who study tumours than are published by the vast majority of researchers who study cell lines.

So using cell lines seems to make a lot of sense. However, in order for a cell to adapt to life in a petri dish, it has to change, at a very fundamental level. That change makes the cell very different from a normal tumour cell. It displays very different characteristics, so the changes invalidate the results gained from research on cell lines. The information gained applies to cell lines – but does not apply to real, living cancer cells, in real, living tumours, in real, living people.

How different are cells in vitro *from cells* in vivo?
Dermer points out a number of differences. Firstly, cancer cells in the body are genetically stable, with fixed characteristics. A breast cancer cell that metastasises in the lung five years later will be identical to the original breast tumour cells. In contrast, cells in cell lines are notably unstable at the chromosomal level. The number and structure of the chromosomes in the cells change in a random way over time. Scientists working with such cells assume that the genetic instability derives from the original breast cancer cell. Pathologists know that's not true.

Another important difference is that cancer tumour cells taken from the body have clear sex chromosomes; cells in cell lines commonly lose these chromosomes. A third difference is that when fresh from a living person, a breast cancer cell is very different from a lung cancer cell, which is different from a rectal cancer cell, etc.; in cell lines, they are indistinguishable. This had a costly result.

111

For a decade or more, many scientists who believed they were studying prostate cancer cells, liver cancer cells or bladder tumour cells were actually studying the HeLa line of cells. Contamination had occurred, and the HeLa line is a particularly dominating cell line. If a cell from HeLa gets into a petri dish containing cells from another line, it quickly colonises the dish and annihilates the other cells. This is what had happened at a number of institutes; it went unnoticed because there was nothing to distinguish one cell line from another. It was only when the weight of anomalous results became apparent over a period of over ten years that the problem was discovered. It may be that this contamination continues, yet as long as papers are accepted for publication, nothing else matters – except that the possibility of a cure remains a mirage, and large numbers of people will continue to die.

Scientists and pathologists
Pathologists' knowledge is dependable, because it is based on the examination of fresh living tumours. Experimental cancer researchers know something else. But what they know is not necessarily applicable – and very likely wholly inapplicable – to human cancer. Pathologists and laboratory cancer experimenters, unfortunately, occupy different scientific worlds. Dr Dermer's comment is that: 'The cancer research community is almost devoid of people who understand human cancer.'

For those who place their hopes on cancer research, this flaw is a major obstacle to success. Recently, there has been a push by women's groups for more research specifically on breast cancer. We can now understand why breast cancer – or any other specific cancer – has not received much specific research. After all, even though an anti-cancer agent is found to have an effect on a supposedly specific cancer cell in the laboratory, it is not credited with being an agent against a specific cancer type until the results of the phase 2 clinical trials have been evaluated. The lobbying groups should push very specifically for research by pathologists.

FLAW TWO
If we turn to animal studies, there appears to be a great deal we can learn. They are based on a simple premise: that all

mammals share a great many physical similarities, and what is true for one species has an increased chance of being true for another. So far so good. The problem is that there are substances that are seriously toxic for rats that have no effect on mice. There are viruses that will devastate man, which are quite innocuous for other primates – HIV being one. Malaria is another. Almost every ape and monkey has its own susceptibilities to a different type of malarial parasite – but few species share susceptibilities with each other. In short, what is true for rats and mice has no necessarily predictive value for man.

FLAW THREE
Medical science has built a cult around the specific test of the human phase of the double-blind clinical trial. Nothing else can replace this experimental procedure and hope to achieve acceptance. The reason for its status is that it is assumed to provide irrefutable results. But is this true? Can we rely on the results gained from clinical trials?

To answer this question, I am going to compare two trials that were conducted to see if vitamin C was an effective agent in the fight against cancer. One of the trials was not double-blind, though it was a controlled study, conducted by the famous vitamin C protagonist, Linus Pauling. The other was a double-blind clinical trial conducted by Dr Charles Moertel, a noted opponent of vitamin C. The trials came up with very different results. The former showed that vitamin C had the power in some cases to cure terminal cancer patients, and for many others to extend their lives. The latter showed that it had no effect.

The Pauling trial was conducted in cooperation with Dr Ewan Cameron at Vale of Leven Hospital in Scotland. Cameron, like Pauling, believed in the efficacy of vitamin C, so he could not ethically refuse to give it to any of his patients for the purposes of a clinical trial. However, he reasoned that as the other doctors at the hospital did not share his views, he could simply compare his vitamin C taking patients with the patients being seen by others. In addition, he asked another doctor to compare his patients against 1,000 past patients, matched by age and disease, who had already received treatment.

Because the trial was not double-blind, the normal

demeanour of the presiding doctor ceased to be a factor. Both Cameron and Pauling made a point of encouraging their patients to feel hopeful about the potential for a cure. The result was very positive. A number of these patients were still alive ten years later, compared with none from any of the other groups.

The Mayo Clinic trial by Dr Moertel was, however, a true double-blind trial conducted by doctors sceptical of the value of the substance they were testing – and with patients who had no idea what they were taking. The doctor-patient interaction was made bland and non-psychologically supportive, in order to rule out the placebo effect (the effect, which has been clearly demonstrated in a wide range of circumstances, where people are cured despite taking pills of no medical value).[7]

So, in the Cameron-Pauling trial, the patients became involved – they bought into it. Doctors and patients were partners, fighting for the same cause. In the Mayo Clinic trial, on the other hand, the doctors didn't even know what they were testing and their patients, too, were deliberately kept in the dark. Doctors remained aloof, patients passive. We can therefore assume that the patients in Cameron-Pauling's test felt better about their situation. This 'feeling good' response may have had a critical importance, as we can see from the following.

It has been argued by Hans Selye, in a book called *The Stress of Life*, that the body goes through three stages in responding to stress:

1. Alarm reaction
2. Stage of resistance
3. Stage of exhaustion.

Most terminal cancer patients are in the final stage. Stages 1 and 3 are typified by over-production of corticoid hormones. Corticoids are stress hormones, and they depress the immune system. This explains the link between stress and illness. They make the body feel bad, to tell the mind that it is time to take a rest. In Stage 2, corticoid hormone levels are normal.

Now, vitamin C has among its many functions the regulation of the production of corticoid hormones. So, in

Stages 1 and 3, the vitamin C intake may be used to produce corticoid hormones rather than go to the aid of the immune system. It may, therefore, have no protective value to the patient – indeed, it may hasten death. The only way to make it valuable is to force the patient back from the stage of exhaustion into the stage of resistance. This has to be done by psychological means: the emotions reflect the physiological status of the body and, similarly, the physiology reflects the emotional status of the body. Happy, involved people are resisting. Tired, frustrated, depersonalised people are exhausted. Hopeful patients live, hopeless patients die.

And so, double-blind studies that deliberately keep patients in a state of uncertainty and helplessness, that see patients as mechanical objects not as active biological beings, cannot detect the value of chemicals that to be effective depend on the patient's own psychological attitude. That is the flaw.

FLAW FOUR

There are flaws of omission as well as of commission. The focus of attention is on the cancer cell – not on the person who has cancer. The bio-chemical terrain in which the cancer cell develops is hardly considered. If we believe that such a cell arrives in the body as an act of God, with no bio-chemical origin, this might make sense. This is one of the dividing lines between orthodox and alternative medicine. Orthodox researchers focus on the problem in its most reduced state – the chemicals in the cell. Alternative researchers look at the whole of the person's body, and seek to determine what is different about that body. As a result, they have found that vitamin C and Omega 3 oils, for example, are deficient in people with cancer. By restoring the balance, they claim to obtain good results. As it is not in the medical mainstream, however, this research gets little funding.

To put this another way, let us take an analogy. The modern scientific cancer researcher is in the position of a Martian who, seeking to understand the game of tennis, approaches the task by minutely analysing a tennis ball. He may come up with fascinating information on the performance potential of the ball and the industrial processes required to produce it – but this will not lead to any real understanding of tennis as a game.

FLAW FIVE

Clinical trials are a cumbersome method of progressing from one truth to another. Ultimately, they require vast resources of time, effort, people and money. If we were to depend entirely on clinical trials, scientific progress would slow to a snail's pace. Problems are subjected to a reductive analysis to ensure that all possible variations are controlled, and that any result that emerges can have only one cause – and the means of action of that cause are clear. Requirements such as these enable science to take leave of common sense.

There are other requirements that have to be satisfied before and during the human phase clinical trials. One of these is that the exact means by which the drug achieves its effect has to be described. Some years ago, scientists at the University of Texas had successful results using Chinese herbs against cancer. The project director was quoted as saying, 'We have something that works, or at least seems to. Our problem, however, is that *we do not know why or how it works*, and until we do, we cannot develop this as a modern medicine.'

So, these Chinese herbs are kept away from patients, despite the scientific evidence that they work. Is this a sane way to go about the management of our health? As consumers of doctors' work, we are entitled to ask this question. Clearly the questions not being applied to the problem are: what is the risk involved, and what is the potential benefit?

If 'proof' is the only acceptable standard, then there is no reason for assuming that smoking causes cancer. The association of tobacco with cancer is statistical. No proof of a classical nature exists – yet 99.99 per cent of scientists believe that smoking causes cancer. Thalidomide was withdrawn from the market – while there was no proof that it caused birth defects, there is no doubt that thalidomide caused those defects. So when doctors and scientists insist on the necessity of *proof*, they are being seriously misleading. Perhaps we need proof that the concept of 'proof' is useful . . .

116

FLAW SIX

Even the results of clinical trials cannot be accepted uncritically. As Dr Steven Rosenberg, Chief of Surgery at the US National Cancer Institute, says: 'I think as many as thirty per cent of scientific articles contain results or conclusions that are wrong and are not reproducible. A good many more stretch their conclusions far beyond what their evidence will support.' It is Dr Rosenberg's view that 'not all people who do science are scientists'; that much depends on the subjective judgement of the investigator – so, ultimately, scientists like himself will tend to distrust all information that doesn't come from a respected source.

FLAW SEVEN

They have not come up with a cure for cancer. As one patient, Hazel Thornton, puts it: 'There is much rejoicing for small advances, but I believe we should be asking, is this activity leading us to finding a cure, and why do these treatments not work and why, in spite of these treatments, is the death rate still so high?'

Control of research by drug companies

One point of view is that pharmaceutical companies have no desire to find a cancer cure – unless it is a cure they can profit from. It doesn't take much cynicism to see the validity of this argument. What industry will support the means by which its own profits are threatened? On the contrary, it is very much in the pharmaceutical industry's interests to impede such work. The most benign way in which this can be done is simply to starve it of funds. In this way, interesting but unprofitable possibilities are sidelined in favour of research into patentable drugs.

Most cancer research is conducted under the umbrella of one or other of the pharmaceutical companies. They provide much of the financing and the means by which a drug can be developed. If their search for a pharmaceutical cure is fundamentally flawed, then all the money put into this kind of research will be wasted. The industry is very happy with the current situation, as the profit margins on the anti-cancer drugs they are currently marketing are very fat. Cancer is good for profits. 'The production of non-patented drugs will give only moderate profits, while the production of patented drugs will give abnormally high profits. Drug manufacturers have attempted, therefore, by every conceivable means to divert the market into the sale of high-profit patented drugs.' (Medical Committee for Human Rights, quoted in Moss, 1982)

If you doubt the influence of the drug companies, look at who is on the controlling boards of the largest cancer research institutions. In the US, it is not uncommon for senior officers retiring from regulatory bodies such as the FDA (Food and Drug Administration) to be given directorships on the boards of the drug companies. So, commercial interests and their influence in the halls of power must be accepted as one of the problems to be overcome by someone seeking acceptance for a new idea.

Scientific status
Commercial interests are not the only obstacles. Another relates to the status of the person demonstrating the proof, or the institution where the work is undertaken. We can see this clearly if we consider the following argument. It seems sensible to say that results emerge from effort, and that the greater the effort, the greater the results will be. If we follow this logic, then we can also argue that the greater the amount of money we spend on a project, the greater the amount of effort that will result. Therefore the places attracting the largest amounts of research money must be the places where the greatest scientific advances will take place. And since those institutes will also be where the scientists with the best reputations will be employed – because their presence attracts research funding – we have a tidy and comfortable picture of scientific eminence and scientific breakthrough walking hand-in-hand.

Conversely, a poorly funded individual of little eminence cannot be expected to achieve much. Certainly, such a person cannot be expected to solve problems that elude the great minds supported by access to large resources. As a result of this and related – perhaps unconscious – prejudices, established bodies will not accept any 'proof' simply because it has been demonstrated. They will, instead, be highly suspicious of any evidence that does not come from certain accepted sources.

This is quite explicitly stated by Dr Robert Harris of the

Imperial Cancer Research Fund, who rejected the value of the work of Dr Joseph Issels: 'But you must remember that millions of pounds are spent on cancer research every year, and you can't expect anybody in this field to seriously believe that somewhere in Bavaria there is a man who's got hold of something which has escaped the rest of us.' (It was Issels' work that led Penny Brohn to set up the Bristol Cancer Help Centre.) However, there appears to be a consistent pattern where this sort of individual, either through rigorously logical reasoning, great genius, bold experimentation, rare opportunity or plain dumb luck, does indeed find the answer – often only to be ridiculed or ignored by the great.

The most famous case in medical history concerns a Dr Ignaz Semmelweiss. It was in a Viennese hospital, in 1848, that Semmelweiss's attention was drawn to a curious fact. There were two maternity wards in the hospital, one attended by doctors and the other by midwives. Semmelweiss discovered that women patients, who should have been clamouring for the attentions of the doctors, were seeking admission to the other ward. There were two possible reasons for this. Either it was a matter of modesty or ill-informed nonsense – as the professors insisted – or the women's reason that fewer died in the midwives' ward had some merit.

To determine the matter, Semmelweiss studied the records and observed events in person. The results were clear. The women patients were right: a great many of those in the doctors' ward died of puerperal fever; relatively few from the midwives' ward did so. What could account for this? Semmelweiss saw that the main difference was that the midwives washed their hands, while the doctors did not. Worse, when not attending to their patients, the doctors were in the next room doing post-mortems on those who had died of puerperal fever.

Semmelweiss started to wash his hands, with the result that few of his patients subsequently got puerperal fever. He therefore theorised that some form of invisible contagion was the cause of the disease; at that time, Louis Pasteur had not yet convinced the world of the germ theory of disease. Puerperal fever was common – forty per cent of women giving birth in hospital got it and more than a third of them died.

119

Semmelweiss sought to persuade the other doctors of his findings – but he was a young provincial Hungarian, in the best hospital in Vienna. His views were derided. When he published the results of ten years of observation in 1861, he suffered vicious attacks on his integrity and was forced to flee Vienna.

Semmelweiss couldn't prove he was right. He didn't understand why he was right, but he *was* right. The sad truth is, experts resist change. And as a postscript to this story, it should be noted that it was the patients who first saw the simple truth that medical experts refused to see for several decades longer.

Dr Eugene Robin calls events of this type 'iatroepidemics' – large-scale attacks on public health, caused by doctors. He notes that radical mastectomy and tonsillectomy are two other common unnecessary procedures which resulted, and continue to result, in unnecessary deaths. Robin also lists three uses of radiation which had disastrous results. One was a programme to X-ray children believed to be at risk from enlargement of the thymus gland – a condition known as status thymaticus. A number of these children later developed cancer of the thyroid gland. This case is particularly ironic, because as Dr Robin explains: 'It is now known that the disease never existed.'

Other doctors think radiotherapy will in the future be seen as an iatrogenic episode. Dr Irwin Bross, who tried to investigate the question of whether radiation therapy was iatrogenic, had his research funding cut off by the National Cancer Institute. Bross wrote: 'It is almost impossible to get "peer review" that will accept a study of iatrogenic disease. For thirty years, radiotherapists in this country have been engaged in massive malpractice – which is something a doctor will not say about another doctor.' (Quoted in Moss, 1982)

Conformity

Why is it that simple evident truths – or interesting possibilities – are so hard for the medical profession to accept? One answer is conformity. Medical researchers conform to the same goal: to seek chemotherapeutic agents that will kill cancer (they test over 50,000 substances each year); they conform to the same method – the use of cancer cells that reproduce themselves in petri dishes; they conform in their funding sources – in the US these must be approved by the National Cancer Institute and in the UK by the Medical Research Council. These bodies are run by groups of respected scientists with a shared vision of how the goal of cancer cure will be achieved. Anyone who does not share that goal will not get funding. Indeed, as Dr Gerald Dermer discovered, they will be cold-shouldered. In this way, an entire industry develops a single perception.

Many cancer researchers wish to advance in their chosen careers – to go from working as part of a team, to leading a team, to heading an institute. To do this, they need to publish results. In order to publish, they must persuade their mentors to add their names to their research – only the previously published get subsequently published. Their articles must also receive the go-ahead from colleagues, under the 'peer-review' system. So, they need to know the right people, they need to say the right things. If there are any fundamental flaws in the assumptions, perceptions or methods of research, then these flaws will invalidate the work of the entire industry. The laws of conformity will ensure that everyone is wrong.

If this is true, then the individual working far from these centres and uncluttered by a ruling theoretical orthodoxy is the one most likely to come up with something interesting, something that works. However, such a scientist would not find it easy to inform the world about his discovery, because the same people who fund science are those who validate and publish its results. New discoveries foreign to normal practice tend to be ignored or sidelined. Peer-review journals will not publish papers that go against the prevailing ethos. Conferences will not accept such papers. Research-funding bodies will not provide the necessary funds to continue the work.

The new discovery has to wait in the wings for unconscionable periods of time before it gets accepted – if it ever does. If the researcher attempts to go public by announcing the discovery to the world at large, he or she is vilified. Witness what happened to the two scientists who came up with the idea of cold fusion. In March 1989 Professors Martin Fleishmann and Stanley Pons astonished the scientific world when they announced that they could produce small amounts of useable energy by a cold-fusion nuclear process that occurred in a jar of water at room temperature. Both men are distinguished scientists. After a short honeymoon period the two scientists were the subject of ridicule in the press and rejection by the scientific establishment. Nevertheless, it appears there actually is a real effect, and this is being studied at an increasing number of laboratories. Hysterical claims of fraudulence have given way to something more reflective – it appears there *is* a cold-fusion effect.

Another force working against the development of new ideas is that institutions are highly competitive. If an idea has emerged from a rival institution, there will be a natural attempt to discredit it. If that doesn't work, then it must somehow be taken over. Current research work is a highly prized secret which must not be revealed to the outside world. Failures are buried; successes applauded unduly.

The authoritarian personality
The structure of the scientific and medical professions is very hierarchical, giving great power and authority to those at the top and requiring submissiveness from those below. At the bottom is the patient. Top-down communication dominates. Obedience is assumed and required.

The concept of two opposing personality constructs – authoritarian and democratic – was put forward by psychologists at Berkeley University in California in the late 1940s. Among the characteristics associated with the authoritarian personality are the following:

- a rigid adherence to conventional values.
- a submissive, uncritical attitude towards leaders of the group with which he or she identifies – they are imbued with idealised moral qualities.
- a tendency to be over-sensitive to violations of the conventional moral order – and to react to these violations by condemning, rejecting and punishing people who violate them.
- a tendency to be opposed to subjective feelings, the world of the imagination, and to emotional generosity.
- a tendency to think in rigid categories.
- a preoccupation with power and dominance – leading to the idealisation of, and submission to, power figures.

122

Since doctors and scientists live and thrive in professions that are highly hierarchical and authoritarian, we can assume that they feel comfortable in such a structure. Science writer Richard Milton, author of *Forbidden Science*, thinks this is the case. He believes that scientists with authoritarian personalities will tend to do better in their world than those with democratic personalities.

Milton quotes the case of a postgraduate student in the 1980s seeking to get support from his professor for permission to study hypnosis. The professor refused to allow it, on the grounds that it was not a respectable field for research. It was not respectable because there was no serious literature; there was no serious literature because no-one had done any research; and no-one had done any research because it was not a respectable field. Joseph Heller coined the term 'Catch-22' to define this form of circular argument. In this case, a potentially serious study of a subject about which little is known is starved of funds and professional support because it contravenes conventional attitudes.

Compare this with the words of Professor John Huizenga, co-chairman of a committee set up to investigate whether funds should be directed into a new area of research: 'It is seldom, if ever, true that it is advantageous in science to move into a new discipline without a thorough foundation in the basics of that field.' This conservative caution may be viewed as the relatively benign face of a potentially malign force. It is one thing not to favour an unconventional approach or subject, it is quite another to root out dissent – scientific or social.

Yet the medical and scientific professions have shown that they are prepared, in certain circumstances, to go to great lengths to root out both dissidence and difference. The rise of Nazism in Germany, for example, would not have been possible without the support of the medical and scientific communities. Robert Jay Lifton studied this, reporting his findings in *The Nazi Doctors: Medical Killing and the Psychology of Genocide*. In the introduction to this book, Lifton says: 'When we turn to the Nazi doctor's role in Auschwitz, it was not the experiments that were most significant. Rather it was his participation in the killing process – indeed his supervision of Auschwitz mass murder from beginning to end. This aspect of Nazi medical behaviour has escaped full recognition.'

The point here is not to point the finger of blame at the present medical profession for the mass murder in Nazi Germany; rather, it is to demonstrate that we are discussing a valid concept that has a profound influence on the medical and scientific professions. Russian doctors sent dissidents to mental hospitals; American doctors lobotomised the mentally ill. In many countries where capital punishment is carried out, doctors are required to be present. It is also common, in countries where it is institutionalised, for doctors to be present during police torture sessions to assess whether it is safe to continue with the torture.

These are extremely painful facts. Perhaps they can be dismissed by saying that they apply to other places and other times. Yet they do establish a general tendency – doctors like to be in charge. As Dr Steven Rosenberg says: 'Too many doctors are comfortable dealing with patients only when they can assume an air of unquestioned authority. Surgeons tend to be particularly authoritative.'

Some research has been done on medical students and their attitude to authority. First and second year medical students have a strong sense of ethical sensitivity, but this deteriorates as they progress through the next three years of their medical studies.

All this is very worrying, and has consequences in the present. The medical profession has persevered for twenty-five to thirty years with a treatment – chemotherapy – that they know doesn't work for the majority of cancers, yet they still give it. And a significant percentage of patients die from this chemotherapy. Yet there is no debate as to its merits. It appears that the senior oncology consultants are wedded to the hope that somehow something will emerge from chemotherapy. This being so, junior members of their teams will not wish to be seen to be out of step. How, then, is change going to occur? How are we to awaken the medical profession from their dream? This can only be done if patients are allowed to become properly informed, and discussion of their treatments is allowed to flourish in a wider arena. This is something, however, that the British medical establishment strongly resists. The British press seemingly acquiesces to this arrangement as well.

Research as a game

Then there is the theory that medical research is like a game, a theory argued by Dr Ashley Conway in an article published in the magazine *Complementary Medicine*. First he distinguished between two types of expert. The Type 1 expert is like an engineer. He knows how to do something useful. If there is a problem he seeks to solve it. When he has solved it, he moves on. The Type 2 expert doesn't know how to solve problems – he simply knows a lot. Dr David Horrobin, who first proposed this distinction, suggests that the area of cancer research is dominated by Type 2 experts. As a result it has got nowhere.

Ashley Conway explains the incentives of turning research into a game. It allows for status recognition within a hierarchical system which has developed rules for how that status can be acquired. It also provides security: 'You know where you are with the Game – it reduces uncertainty, maintains equilibrium, blocks intimacy and keeps an emotional distance which achieves the important effect of making people predictable. The Game enables the Type 2 expert to avoid taking risks and therefore to avoid being wrong.'

Not all researchers are Type 2 experts – but the majority, Conway argues, are. And what happens if a Type 1 expert comes along and solves a problem? One defence is simply to find a flaw in a minor detail and then to dismiss the whole on that basis.

The politics of cancer

The medical profession is socially and politically powerful. The scientific community is entrenched, competitive and defensive. The drug companies wield a great deal of financial clout. Together, they are a formidable social force.

A war has waged in America for several decades between this orthodox establishment on the one side, and proponents of alternative or complementary medicines on the other, a war that is spilling over to Britain. The details are too long and complex to go into in this book. Anyone seeking a good account of its impact in Britain should read *Dirty Medicine* by Martin Walker,[8] which describes the work of a self-proclaimed 'quack-busting' organisation called The Campaign Against Health Fraud and the way it has attempted (very often successfully) to influence the practice of non-orthodox medicine in Britain.

The Campaign Against Health Fraud is just one manifestation of a desire to impose the orthodox version of medicine on the British people and to eliminate all the others. Even before the campaign reached the UK, there was a concerted effort by the medical authorities to keep cancer treatments within the orthodox fold. Indeed this has long been enshrined in British law. Anyone may treat anyone else for flu or even AIDS, but the non-medically qualified person who treats another person's cancer is breaking the law.

Whether or not The Campaign Against Health Fraud is itself responsible, the war against alternative thought has intensified in recent years. The means used are smear campaigns and outright harassment. The bad publicity given to the Bristol Cancer Help Centre in 1990 – when it was alleged that life expectancy of patients at the centre was significantly lower than for those undergoing standard treatments – was an example of the way in which this happens.

The accusation was later shown to be wrong, but it was given wide publicity by a press seemingly delighted to dish the dirt.

Harassment of alternative practitioners and those associated with unorthodox ideas has also occurred. Dr Stephen Davies, a leading British nutritional doctor, has had break-ins at his laboratory, the main target appearing to be his computer data-base – an item of interest to no ordinary thief. This is not an isolated incident. Vitamin manufacturers have been similarly harassed. Such accusations may seem paranoid, yet if even half the things Walker itemises in *Dirty Medicine* are true, then something highly suspect is certainly happening.

Then there is the manipulation of the medical authorities. Over the last ten years, a number of substances that were widely available and generally seen as safe have been taken off the market. One such is niacin. This B vitamin remains legal in the US and most other countries. It is good for the liver and a proven mood lifter. It is now only available in British high streets in combination B complex supplements. What *is* happening in Britain?

Whatever it is, the same thing is happening in Europe. The French, Spanish and Greek governments are pressing the European Union to classify vitamin supplements greater than 1.5 times the RDA (Recommended Daily Allowance) as medicines. This would require them to go through expensive drug-licensing procedures. At one stroke, this could wipe out the dietary supplements business. Only intense lobbying by consumer pressure groups like Consumers for Health Choice prevented this decision from going through in 1992. But the pressure remains. In the US, this war is also being waged, although the pro-vitamin groups appear to have won in most states.

The politics of medicine are as vicious as politics in any other arena of endeavour.

'Unproven therapies'
One of the key concepts in the dispute between orthodox and alternative medicine is the concept of proof. The idea is generally put forward that orthodox methods of treating cancer are 'proven', and that all others are 'unproven'. We have already seen that most orthodox methods are unproven

by any standard. However, the term 'unproven therapies' is used by the American Cancer Society (ACS) to label methods of treatment which it opposes. It is used in much the same way that the word 'Communist' was used by US Senator McCarthy in the 1950s – as a slur.

'Unproven' means simply that no proof has been obtained. It does not mean that a therapy's effectiveness has been *dis*proved. Yet many writers who put forward the establishment view appear to think that it does. They also confuse the words 'evidence' and 'proof'. We may accept that stringent standards have to be satisfied before *proof* is established – but along the way we collect evidence, through tests. These tests must follow accepted scientific procedures. It is common, therefore, to have scientific evidence without necessarily having scientific proof.

The scientific requirements of disproof should be as stringent as the requirements of proof. Yet, despite this, of the therapies listed as 'unproven' by the ACS, almost half arrived there without any investigation being undertaken. There is something curious and indeed unacceptable about the speed with which therapies are rejected. Why is this happening? What is the agenda of the people rejecting them? These are valid questions which need to be answered. Yet there appears to be little desire among those working in the field of cancer research, or medical doctors practising in the leading hospitals of North America and Europe, to demand an answer or to challenge these rejections.

One former official of the American Cancer Society, Pat McGrady, has written:

[The American cancer establishment] has turned the terror of [cancer] to its own ends in seeking more and more contributions from a frightened public and appropriations from a concerned Congress. Still, undismayed by the futility of funds dumped into the bottomless pit of its 'proven' methods, it remains adamant in refusing to investigate 'unproven' methods.

Every book written from a staunchly orthodox stance contains warnings to patients that they should not entertain any thoughts of going down the route of 'unproven' therapies. According to an ACS pamphlet: 'Keep in mind that accepted medical treatment for your cancer is the best *scientifically tested* treatment. The best way to determine whether a treatment is proven or unproven is to ask your family doctor. Doctors rely on scientific proof before they use a treatment. Unproven methods lack such proof.'

Other warnings suggest that 'unproven' methods can cause harm, either directly or indirectly, by seducing patients from proper treatments. Dr Errol Friedberg is so concerned to dissuade the potentially errant patient that he produces the ultimate argument: 'Even if the "treatments" are not in themselves harmful, a serious consequence of their use, and one that is insufficiently recognised by cancer patients and their families, is that *those who use them are wasting valuable time*' (his italics). (Friedberg, 1992) Patients are wasting time that should be used in continuing 'accepted' forms of cancer treatment, and time that should be spent getting used to dying . . .

Clearly, Dr Friedberg assumes that unproven remedies are necessarily ineffective. This is, as we have seen, an unscientific position to take. By having a list of unproven therapies, and by using it as a blacklist to stop further funding, we have a self-fulfilling prophecy. The therapies are unproven because there is no institutional will to seek proof. There is, instead, a will to *prevent* such proof being established. One of the rules of the game is that disproof is assumed. Another rule is that anyone who proposes, or uses, an unorthodox approach has to be slandered as a quack and/or a charlatan.

Underlying the name-calling is a profoundly false assumption. It is one thing to say that a doctor needs scientific proof that a drug is effective – a point that is itself debatable. It is quite another to demand this of patients. Patients don't necessarily need proof – not when the price of that proof is so high. Anecdotal evidence is quite sufficient for most aspects of life. If Mr Brown took substance 'X' and was cured, and Mrs Smith took substance 'X' and was cured of the same thing, you can bet your bottom dollar I will also try 'X' if the need arises. I wouldn't think of waiting thirty or a hundred years for science to get its act together to prove that it worked.

129

Are we missing opportunities?

One of the first examples of a proper controlled test was conducted in 1747, on twelve patients suffering from scurvy. Dr James Lind placed all of them on the same diet except for one item – the supposed remedies that he was testing: citrus fruits, cider, vinegar, sea water, a mixture of drugs. He gave each of these remedies to two patients. At the end of six days, the two who had been given citrus fruits were well, while the others were still ill. Lind published these results in 1753.

This was clearly not a double-blind trial – both Lind and the sailors knew exactly what they were receiving. However, it was rational, rigorously carried out and easily repeatable. It therefore has all the hallmarks of classical scientific testing. Yet, as we have just seen, such a test today would carry little weight with the elders of the accrediting committees that govern medical science. The result might be admitted as interesting, but certainly not conclusive. It does not establish, once and for all, proof that lemons cure scurvy. Under current protocols, many more years of testing would be required to establish such proof. Scientists would need to know why lemons cured scurvy. The active ingredient would have to be isolated and then tested on cells in laboratories, in animal studies and then experimentally in human trials using double-blind procedures.

This is where science and common sense start to follow different roads. All this time, doctors would be warning patients not to take any form of unproven treatment – like lemons – for their scurvy. Yet, for the cancer patient, whose life-span has suddenly foreshortened to the near future, these warnings cannot make sense – and to pretend that they do is simply ridiculous.

We should note in passing that sciences such as physics rely on other perfectly acceptable scientific procedures to develop their ideas. Double-blind clinical trials clearly are not the only valid means of proceeding.

As it happened, Dr Lind's demonstration that the answer to scurvy lay in the lemon was not accepted. On the contrary, since fresh fruits and juices were expensive, there were pressures on ship owners and the established authorities not to accept the results. However, eventually, in 1795 – over forty years after Lind published his results – the British

Admiralty ordered a daily ration of fresh lime juice for all hands. As a result, scurvy disappeared from the Royal Navy. The merchant navy, however, was under the control of the Board of Trade. It wasn't until 1865 – 120 years after the original experiment – that the Board passed its own lime-juice regulations.

Putting it all together

We can now appreciate what Linus Pauling meant when he suggested that a fundamental, organisational blindness prevents science and medicine developing except along narrow, well-trodden, safe pathways through the confusing forests of reality.

'The National Cancer Institute is not operated in a way as to favor the discovery of new methods of controlling cancer. In my opinion, the NCI does not know how to carry on research nor how to recognise a new idea.' (Quoted in Moss, 1982) This, then, is the scientific research that is eating most of the money donated to cancer research, the research that, despite an expenditure of thousands of millions of pounds, has not resulted in any fundamental advance in cancer treatment for the last twenty years. 'It is gradually dawning on the donors that for the past twenty years practical benefits have not followed [from medical research]. During that time, there have been no substantial improvements in morbidity or mortality from major disease that can be attributed to public funding of medical research.' (Dr David Horrobin, 1982, quoted by Milton, 1994)

However, we can also see the problem from the orthodox viewpoint. If surgery, radiation and chemotherapy are to be set aside, what can the doctor do to help the cancer patient? The answer appears to be nothing – especially if that doctor rejects all unorthodox approaches. How could the medical establishment address the world and say: we have nothing in our techno-pharmaceutical armoury that is truly effective against cancer. The uproar would be deafening. The courts would overflow with lawsuits. No establishment in its right mind would voluntarily bring such a response down on its own head. In brief, no matter how damaging and ineffective conventional treatments may be, the orthodox medical practitioner must persevere in directing patients down this path.

From this, it follows that the fact that a treatment is offered by a consultant in a leading cancer institute does not indicate that it is necessarily effective. The patient must always ask for proof or evidence of effectiveness. Usually, as with chemotherapy trials, the result may or may not indicate increased survival – by a week or a month, by two per cent or four per cent. Is this worth fighting for if that time is full of suffering?

If doctors are not going to change standard medical practice, then patients must. Every one of us has the right to choose the therapy we wish to have, based on our own understanding of the facts and awareness of our needs, fears, desires and even prejudices. But if patients are to reject one form of treatment, they must have some idea of the options. And there *are* options: in fact there is a dizzying array of options. Many promise exciting results. For the patient with courage, the picture is not bleak.

Part Three

ALTERNATIVE TREATMENTS

The term 'alternative treatments' covers a wide range of approaches. Most of these therapies have as a central concept the idea that cancer is a disease of the whole body and that the tumour is simply a symptom. Once the cause is cleared up, the symptom will disappear of its own accord. Since they tend to concentrate on the whole body, they are referred to as 'holistic' (or 'wholistic'). Alternative treatments may be used in addition to orthodox treatment, or as something to replace orthodox approaches to cancer.

There is little doubt that people have been cured, or had their lives extended or the quality of their lives improved using many, if not all, of these therapies either on their own or in combination with each other. What is hotly debated is whether any of the therapies can claim *consistently* to cure cancer. Certainly, many of these approaches do claim consistency. However, since this consistency is absent from mainstream methods, a lack of proof of consistency is not a fatal criticism.

Few of these approaches have been clinically tested to any great extent, but the anecdotal evidence that supports them is often persuasive. Many of them, indeed, have been put forward by orthodox medical doctors and bio-chemists. And when they have been tested they have often produced exciting results – without causing the damage associated with mainstream methods. Here then is a survey of the wide range of alternative methods that have been proposed as cancer cures.

Vitamins, minerals and supplements

Free radicals and the need for supplements
There are many processes within the body that help us to remain healthy and resistant to disease. Attacking the body are a wide range of enemies: bacteria, viruses, fungi, poisons, etc. In addition, the body is being damaged by the effects of free radicals. These are molecules that have been deprived of an oxygen atom and are therefore hungry for oxygen. They find this in the fats embedded in the walls of normal cells. They therefore have to attack the cell walls to get the oxygen they require. This damages and can even kill the cell. Free radicals are themselves the normal by-product of the body's chemical reactions – particularly those processes involved in eliminating potentially toxic cellular waste materials. The more toxic waste materials there are in the body, the more free radicals are created.

Free radicals are being formed constantly, but their impact is controlled by the body in a number of ways. Free radicals can also be intercepted before they do any harm. Vitamins A, C and E and the mineral selenium are called antioxidants because they help the body to protect itself in this way. They neutralise the free radicals before they reach the cell walls. Vitamin E works synergistically with selenium, and also works with vitamins A and C by protecting them from oxidation.

Vitamins and minerals have other effects as well. They are co-enzymes, which means they act in some way to help enzymes. Every bodily process requires the actions of enzymes, so if the body is to function well, it needs to have a steady source of vitamins and minerals.

Vitamins are of extremely low toxicity. It takes months on extremely high doses before the body begins to react negatively to those that are fat soluble, like vitamins A and

E. This indicates, on its own, that the body welcomes these vitamins. When the body ceases to be able to tolerate them, it almost always creates a sensation of nausea. If you overdose significantly on vitamin A you will turn a bright orange. This should be sufficient warning to desist! There have been a few – perhaps less than a handful of – cases of people dying from vitamin A poisoning, but the overall position is that far more people have died from complications deriving from aspirin. Also, far more people have died as a result of getting inadequate supplies of vitamins. In fact, if we accept some arguments, most cancers and many forms of heart disease are explicable as the result of inadequate vitamin intake.

What is also interesting is that, even before physical signs detectable by blood tests appear, the mind responds to low levels of vitamins; vitamin B complex deficiency, for example, can lead to mental illnesses. Depression is also a very common response to vitamin C and B deficiency.

Minerals are a slightly different matter. For some there is very little if any toxicity, while for others there are known limits beyond which it would be unwise to go. Details of these are given below.

HOW MUCH DO WE NEED TO TAKE?

There is very little agreement as to how much of any vitamin or mineral we should be taking. British writers tend to be quite conservative, while Americans tend to be much more aggressive. My view is that a risk-benefit analysis favours taking too much rather than too little. People with cancer should be more aggressive than those wishing to provide themselves with some protection. However, very large doses should be built up slowly – and also tapered off slowly.

INDIVIDUALS VARY IN THEIR NEEDS

The RDA (Recommended Daily Allowance) for most vitamins and minerals is extremely low. The term RDA – which in the US has been replaced by the term Reference Daily Intake (RDI), without any change in values – is a measure of the *minimum* amount an *average* person should take. But who is an average person? To be 'average' means to have the characteristics shared by ninety-five per cent of the population. If 500 characteristics were independently inherited, then mathematicians calculate there is only a three per cent chance that even one person in the whole world is completely normal on all 500 characteristics. Since the number of independently variable characteristics is a hundred thousand or more, the inescapable conclusion is that no single human being is 'average', or, therefore, 'normal'.

Taking note of Linus Pauling's observation that there is a wide spectrum of bio-chemical individuality, it may be that some people are suffering deficiencies even though they are receiving much higher than RDA intakes. Modern nutritionists now use another term – ODA (Optimal Daily Allowance). There is some variation as to what constitutes an ODA level, but in all cases it is significantly higher than the RDA.

WILL A MULTI-VITAMIN AND MINERAL STRATEGY PROVIDE A CURE?

There is no one hundred per cent cure. But a study by Albert Hoffer and Linus Pauling compared two groups of cancer patients. Those who continued eating as before had an average life expectancy of just under six months. Those who changed their diets and took high dose multi-vitamin and mineral supplements had an average life expectancy of six years. Women with cancers of the breast, ovaries and cervix did better, averaging ten years. This suggests that whatever else you do, you are well advised to take large doses of vitamins and minerals.[9]

Vitamin C

For anyone seeking to prevent or survive cancer, large doses of vitamin C are highly recommended. However, before starting such a regime, read this section carefully.

THE VITAMIN C CONTROVERSY: SCIENCE AND POLITICS

This controversy is one of the best publicised and most fiercely argued in the annals of non-orthodox cancer treatments. Vitamin C's most famous proponent was Linus Pauling, a double Nobel prize winner (for chemistry, and for peace). Dr Pauling believed that daily 'megadoses' of vitamin C could prevent cancer – and cure it. The 1994 *Independent* obituary of him ended with these words: 'His theories on vitamin C have now been largely discredited.' This is not, in fact, true.

Pauling wrote two books putting forward the evidence in support of vitamin C, *Vitamin C and the Common Cold* and *How to Live Longer and Feel Better*. In them he quoted extensive experimental support for his conclusion that vitamin C has a general anti-viral effect, which protects against any virus – including influenza, polio, hepatitis, mononucleosis and herpes. In addition, he wrote that: 'Good intakes of vitamin C and other vitamins can improve your general health in such a way as to increase your enjoyment of life and can help in controlling heart disease, cancer and other diseases and in slowing down the process of ageing.'

So what theory, evidence or proof did Pauling put forward to substantiate this claim? Firstly, he pointed out that patients with cancer usually have very low concentrations of vitamin C in the blood plasma and leucocytes. This lack prevents the leucocytes from doing their job of engulfing and digesting bacteria and other foreign cells, including malignant cells, in the body. He believed it was reasonable to suppose that the low level of vitamin C indicated that it was being used up in the effort to control the disease. By giving patients a larger amount of vitamin C, their bodily defences should therefore be strengthened.

This, then, was his starting point. He also took note of an interesting case described by a Dr Greer in 1954. This case involved an elderly executive of an oil company who had leukaemia, chronic heart disease and alcoholic cirrhosis of the liver. After having some teeth extracted, he was advised to take vitamin C – its healing effect on gums is well known. The man immediately began to take very large doses (25–42 grams a day). On two occasions, his doctor insisted that he stop taking so much vitamin C. When he stopped, he immediately had problems with his spleen and liver and his leukaemia symptoms returned, all of these rapidly disappearing once he returned to his vitamin C regime. He eventually died of heart disease, but his cancer had been controlled throughout the time he took the vitamin C.

Further evidence came from epidemiological studies that showed higher cancer incidence among people whose vegetable and vitamin C intakes were low.

Pauling then established a professional relationship with

the Scottish doctor, Ewan Cameron. Cameron had come to the same conclusion by another route. His starting point was the known fact that malignant tumours produce an enzyme, hyaluronidase, that attacks the intercellular cement of the surrounding healthy tissues. This weakens the cement to such an extent that the cancer is able to invade. Cameron suggested that one way of defending against the disease might therefore be to strengthen the intercellular cement. Since vitamin C is known to be involved in the synthesis of collagen – the material of which the intercellular cement is composed – high doses of vitamin C should strengthen these defences by allowing faster synthesis, thereby protecting against the spread and growth of a tumour.

Cameron and Pauling started to experiment with vitamin C on terminal cancer patients at Vale of Leven Hospital in Scotland over the next few years. The results were very exciting. The patients treated with a daily 10 grams of sodium ascorbate had a survival time 4.2 times longer than patients who did not take such large doses. A significant percentage of the 'terminally ill' patients went on to long-term survival. In short, for some patients, vitamin C cured their cancer.

One would have expected the cancer associations to have been leaping over themselves to replicate the results. Nothing could be further from the truth. Pauling took the results back to the National Cancer Institute in America, who were, they said, only interested in animal studies. But when Pauling applied for grants to conduct animal-based research, he was turned down eight times. Eventually, he publicised what was happening by publishing an advertisement in the *Wall Street Journal* seeking private donations to help him continue his research.

Eventually, pressure built up and the Mayo Clinic was asked to conduct clinical trials of vitamin C. One of these was conducted by Dr Moertel in 1985. His conclusion, which was widely reported in the press, was that there was no evidence that vitamin C had any beneficial effect on cancer patients. Pauling was severely critical of the conduct of this trial: '[Moertel] suppressed the fact that the vitamin C patients were not receiving vitamin C when they died and had not received any for a long time (median 10.5 months). [This misrepresentation] has done great harm. Cancer patients have informed us that they are stopping their vitamin C because of [these] "negative results".'

Why was the US National Cancer Institute so keen to ally itself to a negative result for vitamin C and so slow to support positive findings? Critics point to the fact that the pharmaceutical industry is well represented in the committees and sub-committees of the leading cancer-related institutions. If it were ever found that vitamin C was a powerful anti-cancer agent, then the pharmaceutical companies could say goodbye to their lucrative business. Others deride such thinking as paranoid. Doctors too get cancer, they say, and they would be mad to turn their backs on any substance that had a reasonable chance of curing the disease. Perhaps – but since the disputed Mayo Clinic trial there has been no proper study of the effects of vitamin C, while more and more doctors are themselves taking large doses of this vitamin.

HOW MUCH VITAMIN C DO WE NEED?

Clearly, vitamin C has a wide range of functions within the body and is an important nutrient. The official RDA for vitamin C is 60 mg per day. Most people assume that the RDA is the average intake to aim for, or an amount which should not be exceeded. In fact, this is wrong. 60 mg a day is the quantity needed to ensure we do not get deficiency diseases like scurvy. So the RDA is a *minimum* recommendation. Vitamin C is a food substance, or nutrient. Applied to food intake as a whole, does it make sense to take in only the amount of nourishment that will prevent us dying of starvation? Frankly, this seems an absurd argument.

Once we have established that the RDA is a minimum amount, we need to find out the ODA, which will presumably be somewhere between the minimum and the maximum amount. But what is the maximum? This will clearly be that amount that will lead to toxicity or ill-health. Taking this as a guideline, we discover an interesting fact: there is no toxic level of vitamin C. (One suggestion that it could lead to kidney stones has not had any experimental support.)

There are two reasons for this lack of toxicity. Firstly, the body welcomes vitamin C in large quantities. Secondly, if the body gets more vitamin C than it can handle at any one time, it dumps the excess by causing diarrhoea, which stops as soon as vitamin C levels become manageable again. This diarrhoea-causing amount varies from person to person. Known as the bowel-tolerance level, it will normally be in the region of 10–20 grams a day for a healthy adult, but it will increase sharply to 30–60 grams, or even more, if there is a viral infection. Going back to Pauling's argument, this suggests that the body is capable of using more vitamin C at times of ill-health, leading to the conclusion that the body is using the vitamin to fight the illness. So one measure of the ODA would be an amount slightly less than the bowel-tolerance level.

We can approach this matter from another angle. Humans are one of a small group of animals, including other apes, that don't produce vitamin C in their bodies. For us, vitamin C has to be taken in from outside, i.e. in food. Most mammals, however, manufacture vitamin C in their livers through the action of a particular enzyme – and they do so in large quantities. A goat, for example, produces approximately 13 grams ($\frac{1}{2}$ oz) a day per 70 kg (155 lb) of body weight, but when stressed it will produce up to 100 grams ($3\frac{1}{2}$ oz) or more. Mice produce 275 mg of vitamin C per kg ($2\frac{1}{4}$ lb) of body weight a day under normal conditions. (A mouse the size of a 70 kg man would therefore be producing 19 grams/$\frac{3}{4}$ oz a day.) These amounts can increase tenfold when the animal is under stress.

This is, for me, the clinching evidence that large quantities of vitamin C are the 'normal' levels we should be taking in for optimal health. Firstly, since man is a mammal, he almost certainly needs vitamin C in quantities similar to other mammals of the same size and weight. Secondly, if animals produce more vitamin C when they are under stress, then presumably the vitamin helps the body cope with stress – and illness is a form of physical stress. Interestingly, dogs and cats, which have relatively low vitamin C production capabilities have, after man, the highest cancer rates in the animal kingdom.

So, we can conclude that vitamin C is needed and that there are very good reasons for suggesting that a lot rather than a little is what the doctor ordered (or should be ordering, even if he isn't inclined to). Many people in America and Australia are taking 10 grams (or more) a day just to maintain their health. For children, one expert

141

recommends that they should take 1 gram per year of life; therefore, an eight-year-old could take 8 grams a day.

IS IT REALLY SAFE?
The drug company Hoffman-LaRoche produced a booklet on vitamin safety in Australia. In this booklet, it said: 'Overall, an exhaustive recent review of the scientific data concluded that vitamin C is a safe substance – even with daily megadoses.' (Quoted by Dettman *et al*, 1993) To deal with the argument that large doses of vitamin C merely lead to 'expensive urine' – i.e. to wasted vitamin C – experts have made the following points:

- The urinary system is very prone to infection, and so it makes sense to direct an anti-viral, anti-bacterial agent like vitamin C through this system.
- The presence of vitamin C in the urine does not indicate tissue saturation, which causes diarrhoea. The amount needed to get a urine reading is very much lower than the amount needed to cause diarrhoea.
- The level of vitamin C in the urine is a good indication of the level in the tissues. If urinary levels are low, then the tissue levels will also be low. High levels of excreted vitamin C are indications that the body's defences are in good shape.
- Vitamin C is cheap!

HOW TO TAKE VITAMIN C
Having established its credentials, it is now necessary to explain that there are a number of different forms of vitamin C, and that they are not all equal.

As straight ascorbic acid, it is very acidic and may lead to intense indigestion. In this form it is also difficult to dissolve in water – although, as a suspension, it can be used as a mouth wash. Usually, vitamin C tablets are 'buffered', which means they are in a non-acidic form.

Most pro-vitamin C advocates warn that the calcium ascorbate form may be good for cancer prevention but must not be used when a cancer tumour is present. This is because calcium stimulates the growth of cancer, and so can lead to a faster decline in the patient's condition. Unfortunately, most on-the-shelf vitamin C pills are calcium ascorbate. A

142

relatively new form of calcium ascorbate – called Ester C – is now on the market. It claims to be four times more effective than normal vitamin C, measured by its length of retention in the body and its bio-availability (its ability to be absorbed usefully by the body). This makes it good for prevention, but remember that it should not be taken by anyone already diagnosed with a tumour.

For cancer patients, sodium ascorbate is the preferred form. This can be prepared at home by mixing pure ascorbic acid and baking soda. The resulting powder can then be taken with any food, e.g. in cereal, on ice-cream, or as a suspension in a drink.

Only an ascorbate salt should be taken intravenously, because ascorbic acid itself damages the veins and tissues into which it is injected. Linus Pauling preferred to take L-ascorbic acid, fine crystals, in orange juice or with a small amount of baking soda. In whatever form, it should, ideally, be divided into a number of equal doses and taken at regular intervals throughout the day. This is to maintain a high average daily level in the tissues.

Vitamin C is best taken with an equal amount of bioflavonoids, commonly found with vitamin C in nature. They are believed to protect vitamin C and to promote its absorption by the body. In combination they are also effective against oral herpes.

Pauling warned that anyone going on a megadose regime of vitamin C to fight a cancer should not start with large doses – there is a danger of the tumour haemorrhaging, which can be fatal. Large doses should be gradually built up over a period of weeks, starting with, say, 3 grams a day and increasing by 2 grams every other day, continuing until the bowel tolerance level has been established. A dose slightly lower than this should then be maintained.

In addition, Pauling warned that you should not abruptly stop taking it – instead the amount should be tapered off. He warned that a sudden stop might result in 'rebound scurvy'. Not everyone believes that this is a danger, but as it may be, it is wise to take precautions.

Lastly, it is important that the cancer patient taking vitamin C should be encouraged and helped to adopt a positive, resisting frame of mind in order to maximise the potential benefits of the vitamin.

Sources: Vitamin C supplements are available at health shops and pharmacies.[10]

SUMMING UP

Until a few months before his death at the age of ninety-three, Linus Pauling was alert and still working. Clearly, he was living proof of the value of the regime he was recommending. Pauling's own recipe for longevity, which he published in 1986, is as follows:

1. Take 6–18 grams of vitamin C every day. Do not miss a single day.
2. Take 400–1,600 iu of vitamin E a day.
3. Take 1–2 high-dosage vitamin B tablets a day.
4. Take 25,000 iu of vitamin A a day.
5. Take a multi-mineral supplement, which should include calcium, iodine, copper, magnesium, manganese, zinc, molybdenum, chromium and selenium, every day.
6. Keep intake of ordinary sugar (including brown sugar and honey) to below 50 lb (22.5 kg) a year.
7. Apart from sugar, eat what you want – but not too much of any one food. Don't get fat.
8. Drink plenty of water.
9. Keep active and exercise, but never excessively over-exert yourself.
10. Drink alcohol only in moderation.
11. Don't smoke.
12. Avoid stress. Work at a job that you like. Be happy with your family.

Vitamin A (and/or beta-carotene)

Beta-carotene is known as the precursor of vitamin A. Vitamin A is obtained from animal sources, while beta-carotene comes from vegetables. Beta-carotene is only changed to vitamin A in the body when it is needed, so vitamin A is best taken in the form of beta-carotene. In that way, any negative effects can be eliminated.

In a controlled study with people who chew betel nut and therefore have a higher incidence of oral cancer, the group who received vitamin A (200,000 iu per week) had a pronounced remission from pre-cancerous lesions and had fewer new lesions. One 1985 study showed that cancer spread was much lower among mice fed with vitamin A supplements. Another study showed that women who took vitamin A during chemotherapy reported a much lower incidence of unpleasant side-effects – no doubt because of its important role for the growth of epithelial tissue. A Finnish study, however, came up with the seemingly odd result that smokers in the high beta-carotene group had a shorter life span than those on a low beta-carotene diet. This study is often produced gleefully by those hostile to supplements, but the fact is, it goes against the grain of all the other studies.

Sources: Active vitamin A is found in fish oils, liver, eggs and dairy products. Yellow vegetables and fruits like mangoes contain beta-carotene. In both forms it is very susceptible to oxidation and can be destroyed by heat and light, so carrot juice has to be freshly pressed and drunk quickly to be effective.

Optimal Daily Allowance: Per day, 10,000–50,000 iu is recommended, though amounts up to 100,000 iu can be taken for extended periods – three to four months – in the case of patients fighting cancer.

Toxicity: Vitamin A may cause birth defects or be toxic to infants, so pregnant and lactating women should keep their intake low (5,000 iu or less). Also women who wish to become pregnant should reduce their vitamin A intake well in advance of conception. Vitamin A is stored in body fat and is not water soluble, so there is the potential for toxicity. However, you need to take at least 100,000 iu daily for a period of months in order to display any signs of toxicity. Beta-carotene, on the other hand, can be given for long periods of time virtually without risk of toxic effects. Signs of toxicity include: yellowing skin, fatigue and nausea, blurred vision and loss of hair.

Vitamin E

Various studies have shown low vitamin E levels in the blood of people with lung, breast, bladder, cervix, and colon or rectal cancers. In a study of mice exposed to cigarette smoke, those supplemented with vitamin E and selenium suffered eight per cent deaths, compared with fifty-one per cent for those fed a diet deficient in these two substances.

145

One study showed that a group of women with the lowest vitamin E levels had five times the risk of breast cancer, compared with a group with the highest vitamin E levels. Some studies have also shown that vitamin E may help to reduce the side-effects of chemotherapy.

Sources: Vitamin E is found in vegetable fats and oils, whole grains and dark green leafy vegetables, nuts and legumes. However, food processing eliminates most of this content. Unrefined or cold-pressed oils are best.

Optimal Daily Allowance: The recommended levels are 200–800 iu per day (some advise up to 1,600 iu per day).

Toxicity: Not advised for those with high blood pressure. However, no toxic effects have been clearly shown for doses below 3,000 iu per day. Signs of toxicity include: nausea, flatulence, headache and fainting.

Vitamin B complex

These vitamins are not all – or even mainly – antioxidants. However, there are some anti-cancer effects. Riboflavin (B2) deficiencies have been shown to lead to high levels of oesophageal (throat) cancer in animals. Vitamin B3 has demonstrated protective properties against pancreatic cancer, and is known to be good for the liver. It has also been shown to increase the effectiveness of radiation treatment. Mice who were given B3 (niacin) showed significantly greater tumour regression as a result of radiation, compared with another group not given niacin. Lastly, niacin is known to have positive effects on mood, so can be taken as an antidepressant.

Vitamin B12 appears to have a strong synergistic relationship with vitamin C. In one animal study in which mice were implanted with tumour cells, only two out of fifty receiving the combination developed tumours. All fifty of the controls developed tumours. However, B12 on its own may have a tumour encouraging effect. A Japanese study shows that large intakes of folate (10–20 mg/milligrams) in combination with 750 mcg (micrograms) of B12 had a very impressive protective effect.

Individual B vitamins should not be taken individually in large doses for any length of time, as this can lead to deficiencies in the other B vitamins – because they compete. The general rule of thumb is that you can take individual B vitamins up to three times their normal value in comparison with the intake of B complex as a whole.

Sources: Widely available in dark green leafy vegetables, beans, brown rice and brewer's yeast, but cooking reduces the bio-availability (or usefulness) of B complex.

Optimal Daily Allowance: B2: 50–500 mg; B3: 50–1,000 mg; B12:100–500 mcg; folic acid: 800–2,400 mcg (with zinc supplementation).

Toxicity: No known toxic effects for B2 and B12, but for B3 (niacin) there is the potential for a flushing or itchy reaction. Folic acid is not associated with any toxic effects.

Vitamin D

This vitamin is necessary for the absorption of calcium. Combined with calcium, it has cancer-protection properties.

Sources: Fish oils are the best source, but otherwise vitamin D is synthesised internally when we expose ourselves to sunlight. People with little exposure to sunlight are at risk of deficiency and should supplement.

Optimal Daily Allowance: 400–600 iu. More for women than men. Older women can take up to 800 iu.

Toxicity: None is known for intakes less than 1,000 iu per day. However, symptoms of overdosing are irreversible and can be fatal – involving calcification of the kidneys and liver.

Selenium

Selenium is needed by all the tissues of the body. Selenium deficiency is quite common, because in many parts of the world the soil is low in this mineral, and the result is that animal and vegetable produce from this land contains very little. People exposed to environmental pollution may become deficient, as selenium is used up fighting the heavy metals. There is very strong evidence that selenium deficiency is implicated in heart disease and cancer – and that these problems can be rectified by adding selenium to the diet in the form of supplements. Vitamin E and selenium work together synergistically – that is, their combined effect is greater than the sum of their effects when taken separately. For our purposes, selenium is known to help protect cells from damage from free radicals. The Japanese take in two to four times more than Americans or Europeans, and their cancer rates are significantly lower.

Optimal Daily Allowance: 200–400 mcg per day.

Toxicity: Anyone taking in more than 2,000 mcg per day may suffer effects such as a garlicky odour in the breath, urine and sweat. Birth defects may also occur with long-term intake at these levels. Long-term intake of 500–750 mcg has not turned up any sign of toxicity in people.

Calcium

As a cancer preventative, calcium appears to be useful. It needs to be taken with vitamin D and magnesium for absorption. For people who already have cancer, however, calcium supplements should be *completely* avoided – silica should be taken instead. Calcium appears to stimulate cancer growth, according to a number of doctors. Max Gerson also believed calcium to be dangerous, blaming a number of cancer deaths on his use of the nutrient.

Even when calcium is desired, not everyone agrees that calcium supplements or a meat and dairy diet are good ways to take it. On the contrary, some people argue that calcium supplements may actually be encouraging the leaching process by which calcium leaves the bones. Calcium, they say, should be taken in vegetable form. Their argument is that milk and meat – the sources of calcium with which we are most familiar – make our systems acidic, and the body releases calcium from our bones to neutralise this effect. In support of this view, some studies have shown that vegetarians have a significantly lower incidence of osteoporosis than meat eaters.

Sources: Seaweeds like kelp, all leafy greens, figs, dates and prunes.

Optimal Daily Allowance: 1,000–1,500 mg per day.

Toxicity: No known toxicity, but take in divided doses to aid absorption along with half as much magnesium and with vitamin D.

Germanium

It is important to stress that there are two forms of this mineral: organic and inorganic. Some cases of kidney failure have occurred with the latter. Inorganic germanium dioxide has also led to kidney failure. However, water-soluble, organic germanium does not have these problems. Indeed, it is considered to have an extremely powerful anti-cancer effect – in addition to its ability to normalise the whole body chemistry.

The discoverer of organic germanium, Dr Kazuhiko Asai, a coal engineer, wrote of the organic germanium that he had synthesised: 'My organic germanium compound has proved effective against all sorts of diseases, including cancers of the lung, bladder, larynx and breast.' He believed the reason for this ability was that germanium enriched the oxygen levels in the body. 'I should say that all diseases are attributable to deficiency of oxygen. The dangers of an oxygen deficiency in the human body cannot be over-emphasised.'

Sources: Medicinal plants, notably shelf fungus (*Trametes cinnabarina*). Garlic and ginseng also contain significant amounts.

Optimal Daily Allowance: None, but recommended dose in case of need: 30–150 mg.

Toxicity: At levels below 500 mg, no toxic effects have been reported. Skin rashes and stool softening have been reported for doses of over 2 grams a day.

Silica
One writer, Klaus Kaufmann, extols the virtues of silica in these words: 'Silicon is the most important element on earth after oxygen. Research has shown that silicic acid, a compound of silicon and water, was one building block of the primary substance from which life was created.'

Silica is the earth's most prevalent mineral and we ingest large amounts of it in the food we eat. It is a necessary component for most of our tissues. It is known that the silica content of heart, kidneys and muscles stays constant throughout life, while that of the skin and thymus gland decreases with age. Not much is known about silica, except that it is very important for bones and for the formation of collagen. It is thought to work in two beneficial ways. Firstly, it strengthens the connective tissues at the cellular level. Secondly, it helps to eliminate harmful substances like uric acid and nicotine from the body.

Some biochemists believe that most of the useable calcium in the body derives from magnesium and silicon –

and that therefore these supplements are more important than calcium for osteoporosis.

There is growing evidence that silica has a vital role to play when it comes to cancer. In the area of Daun in West Germany, there is a very low incidence of the disease, which is attributed to the very high silica content of the local water. One French study has shown that cancer rates drop in areas of high soil silica content, and vice versa. It is known that silica is absent, or present in very low quantities, in people with bone cancer.

Silica is well known for its strength-giving effects on hair and fingernails. Good hair and strong nails are also good general indicators of health. Since the body becomes depleted of silica with old age, there appears to be a good argument for taking silica supplements.

Sources: The best source of organic silica is the plant known as horsetail. Kaufmann recommends that the silica be one hundred per cent pure aqueous extract and derived from spring horsetail – not from any other member of the horsetail family.[11]

Iron

Some believe that iron has the effect of encouraging an already existing tumour, others that it does not have this effect. What is known is that low iron concentrations result in a lowered immune system, with a possibly increased risk of cancer. However, one study seems to indicate that high blood concentrations of iron have the opposite effect, increasing the risk of cancer in men – but the effect on women is unclear.

Anaemia, the well-known iron-deficiency symptom, may not in fact be caused by iron deficiency. It can be caused by a deficiency of vitamin B12 and/or folic acid, as well as by the presence in the bloodstream of drugs or toxins. Therefore, iron does not automatically need to be taken when anaemia is diagnosed.

Sources: Meat, especially liver, eggs, cereals, leafy vegetables, potatoes, fruit and milk.

Optimal Daily Allowance: Men: 15–20 mg; Women: 20–30 mg.

Toxicity: Up to 75 mg can be taken per day with little risk of ill-effects.

Zinc and magnesium

One study published in the *Medical Press* in 1953 – and ever since, largely neglected – showed that an injection of zinc and magnesium ascorbates in aqueous solution had a very profound effect on seven women with terminal cancer of the uterus. Five years later, four of the patients were still alive. In all, 200 terminal cancer patients received the substance; ninety per cent were free from pain within ten days. Many demonstrated tumour regression. In addition to vitamin C, the patients also received a 3 cc injection every other day; each cc of the solution contained 1.5 mg zinc and 0.3 mg magnesium, both complexed with ascorbic acid.

Zinc is well known for its beneficial effect on the thymus gland. Together with magnesium, it appears to act as a very powerful immune system stimulant. This is treatment that any GP could carry out.

Bee pollen

An ounce (or 25 g) of bee pollen each day will, according to naturopath Diane Stein, prevent or delay the development of malignant tumours and help to reduce the size of existing tumours.

Amino acids

Amino acids are the fundamental components of all muscles, organs, glands, body fluids, the enzymes necessary for the body's bio-chemical functioning, the neurotransmitters that take messages to and from the brain and even the nucleus of every cell in the body. They are the molecular bricks from which proteins are built. The body contains something in the region of 50,000 different proteins and 20,000 different enzymes. These are built up by combining twenty-nine known amino acids in different combinations. Each combination is highly specific, and if only one amino acid is missing or present in inadequate quantities the result is that proteins or enzymes are not created, and are therefore not available to the body. The body's functioning becomes impaired.

Eighty per cent of our amino acids are produced by the liver – so a healthy liver is a prerequisite for proper and sufficient amino acid supply. The other twenty per cent comes from diet. The eight amino acids – known as essential amino acids – that must come from our diet are: isoleucine, leucine, lysine, methionine, phenylalanine, threonine, tryptophan and valine. Two others are synthesised in the body from essential amino acids: cysteine from methionine, and tyrosine from phenylalanine.

The value or otherwise of supplementing with amino acids is much disputed. It seems that restriction of specific amino acids helps slow down tumour growth. This would certainly support those who argue for low-calorie diets or fasts as beneficial approaches to cancer treatment. The one clear exception seems to be Glutathione which has shown powerful anti-tumour activity – especially for liver cancer – and is important for various immune system functions and helps protect red blood cells. Other amino acids have shown contradictory effects in a variety of studies with different cancers, and specialist advice is needed for individual cases.

Enzymes

All of the chemical changes inside the body are performed by the action of enzymes. Enzymes are required to digest and decompose all the foods we eat. They enable the gas exchange required for oxygen to move through the membranes of the lungs into the blood system. Enzymes help to stop bleeding and create new cells, which promotes healing. If we are deficient in enzymes, then all the body's processes will start to fail. Enzymes are destroyed at temperatures higher than normal body temperature. All foods that go through a heating process – e.g. canning, freezing – have their enzymes destroyed. Enzymes can only be obtained from fresh food or supplements.

Every chemical process in our body is mediated by enzymes. There are more than 2,700 enzymes in the body – a deficiency in any one will result in a reduced ability to function. Enzymes are therefore of vital importance to health. For cancer prevention and cure, we are concerned with the enzymes that aid digestion. These enable us to digest proteins (proteolytic enzymes) better, to break them down to their amino acid components; to digest fats (lipases); and to decompose carbohydrates (amylases). This explains why the slow and persistent chewing of food helps us to digest food properly – the enzymes have a longer time

152

in which to work on breaking it down to absorbable components. This means more of the food is taken into the body in a form that is capable of being used to support the body's bio-chemical processes.

It is claimed by a number of people that proteolytic enzymes – individually or combined with others – can help to fight or control cancers. The absence of these enzymes may also allow cancer cells to grow. The claims are based on the idea that enzymes:

- promote the body's production of a substance called tumour necrosis factor (TNF), which attacks cancer cells
- directly attack cancer cells
- prevent or diminish metastatic activity, so stopping the cancer cells from spreading.

Studies investigating the effect of enzymes on cancer have been going on for nearly a century. Dr John Beard, a Scottish embryologist at the turn of the century, found that pancreatic enzymes injected directly into tumours restricted their growth. He used enzymes from young lambs, pigs and calves, treating 170 terminally ill patients. They lived longer and in less pain than untreated patients.

Pain relief is one of the major bonuses of enzyme therapy. It is even suggested that the excruciating pain experienced by terminally ill cancer patients can be powerfully alleviated by taking enzymes. These enzymes work synergistically with vitamins A and, more especially, E.

Critics of enzyme therapy say that any enzymes eaten will be destroyed in the digestive tract and therefore cannot enter the body by this route. However, proponents maintain this is not the case. Enzymes, which are themselves large protein molecules, can be ingested through the digestive tract into the blood stream through a process known as pinocytosis. They should be taken on an empty stomach – i.e. thirty minutes before, or ninety minutes after, a meal.

Enzyme therapy is better known and more developed as a cancer therapy in Germany. The most highly regarded enzyme preparations are the Wobe Mugos brand[13]. In Austria, a lumpectomy is generally accompanied by an injection of Wobe Mugos enzymes, rather than radiation.

Sources: Papaya (papain), pineapple (bromelain) and sprouting beans or seeds are high in useful proteolytic enzymes – though all fruits and vegetables contain useful enzymes. The need for food sources to be fresh and raw explains why juices are better than the original vegetable, which often needs to be cooked to be palatable. Pancreatin is an important enzyme that comes from the pancreas. Other important enzymes are contained in extracts from the thymus gland. A simple way to get enzymes in good quantities is to sprout your own mix of beans and to eat or juice them fresh. For further information, read *The Sprouting Book* by Ann Wigmore.

SOD (Superoxide Dismutase)

SOD is a non-toxic enzyme with two very valuable characteristics. Firstly, it has shown anti-cancer activity in its own right, and it appears to be one of the body's natural weapons against tumours. For this reason, most cancer patients show increased levels of SOD in the blood when compared with normal controls. SOD always appears combined with a trace mineral – zinc, copper, etc. Rats injected with copper-bound SOD showed marked benefits, with four doses resulting in seventy-five per cent remission rate. Anyone with cancer should try to get hold of a doctor who will provide this treatment.

SOD also significantly reduces the side-effects of radiation and chemotherapy, without interfering with either. Lipsod, another brand-name SOD product, has been successfully used to treat even long-established fibrosis, reducing it by about a third and softening much of the remainder, resulting in much greater levels of comfort. No other product or treatment is known to have any effect on fibrosis.

Sources: These enzyme products are best delivered by intramuscular injection, using an oral SOD product known as Oxy-5,000 forte.[12] Oral SOD products are sold in health stores, but the concentrations are inadequate for healing purposes. Orgotein is the registered name of a long-lasting form of SOD. (See also Reducing the side-effects of radiation and chemotherapy, page 101.)

To supplement or not to supplement

Among health-conscious people there is a debate as to whether supplements are a good thing. Those who argue

154

against supplements put forward the following views:

- we should be able to get all the nutrients we need from a healthy diet, so rather than take supplements we should concentrate on making sure we eat a properly balanced diet.
- supplements themselves have gone through some form of processing – and therefore suffer from the defects attributed to other processed foods.
- vitamins and minerals work best when they are in organic combinations with other vitamins and minerals; in this form they work synergistically, and so the resulting benefits are maximised.

Those who favour supplements argue as follows:

- we need to take larger quantities of most vitamins and minerals than we can easily find in the food we eat; vitamin C is an obvious example.
- pollution depletes our vitamin resources.
- much of the food we eat has had most of the vital nutrients destroyed by heating during the cooking process.
- we cannot be sure the food we eat is not depleted of vital nutrients by the use of artificial fertilisers and pesticides. In fact, given the wide use of pesticides, it is likely that most vegetables are poor in minerals (pesticides leach minerals from the soils). Since the mineral content of vegetables comes from the soil, diet is unlikely to provide what we need. In the case of animal husbandry, intensive farming techniques combined with the use of antibiotics and hormones make the food a poor source of wholesome nutrition.

The arguments, on both sides of the dispute, are sensible. My own view, however, is that the pro-supplement arguments are stronger (though it is true that there is a great deal of difference in the quality of various supplements) and that you need to find sources of good-quality supplements.[13]

Diet

The idea that food might have something to do with cancer prevention or cure is one that has not always been encouraged by the US National Cancer Institute (NCI): 'There is no diet that prevents cancer in man. Treatment of cancer by diet alone is in the realm of quackery.' (Dr Morris Shinkin, quoted in Moss, 1982) For decades, spokesmen for the leading US cancer institutions poured scorn on those who promoted 'wonder foods'. Yet it is now accepted that a high fibre diet is important for intestinal health. However, nutrition still plays a very minor role in a doctor's education.

This neglect of nutrition is a modern phenomenon. Some 2,500 years ago, Hippocrates said: 'Let food be your medicine and medicine be your food.' A mere 600 years ago, Paracelsus talked of curing cancer by natural means: 'In the hand of the physician, nutrition can be the highest and best remedy.' Unfortunately, he didn't keep statistics . . . The idea that nature does not need to be over-ridden by drugs became derided – and still is by large numbers of doctors. But people are voting with their stomachs, and scientists from the NCI are belatedly finding evidence to support their concerns.

The evidence

One 1994 US study reported a sharp drop in the incidence of colon cancer between 1985 and 1988 – eight per cent for men and eleven per cent for women. 'The most salient risk factor for colorectal cancer is diet.' The authors reported that dietary fat, particularly animal fat, was associated with a high risk, and dietary fibre, particularly insoluble or grain fibre, was associated with low risk. Fruits, vegetables and vitamin D were also seen to have a protective effect, while a sedentary lifestyle and obesity were correlated with a higher incidence of colorectal cancer.

These are very significant findings. Evidence that diet and environmental factors could be the key to all cancers is, of course, implicit in comparisons of cancer rates in different countries. We know it is not genetic, because immigrant families, after a generation or two, develop the cancer profiles of their host countries.

Compare the following:

Age-adjusted death rates per 100,000 population for colon cancer (1988–91)

	Men	Women
USA	16.7	11.4
England and Wales	20.2	13.7
Ireland	23.2	15.1
Scotland	20.6	15.2
Germany	21.1	15.2
Denmark	22.8	17.5
France	17.3	10.3
Spain	13.2	9.2
Italy	15.6	10.3
Greece	6.8	5.5
Japan	15.1	9.7
China	7.9	6.5
Hong Kong	14.8	10.7
Mexico	3.3	3.1
Argentina	13.7	9.3
Chile	7.0	6.0

Source: CA: A Cancer Journal for Clinicians, *American Cancer Society*

The high incidences in northern Europe, dropping as we move to the Mediterranean, and the very low rates in countries where the diet is largely cereals and vegetables, gives a clear indication that the diets of prosperous countries, high in animal fats, are to blame for significant numbers of cancer cases. Wealthy Hong Kong compares badly with neighbouring China. Is this likely to be genetic?

Colon cancer has clear links to food. What about other cancers?

Breast cancer death rates per 100,000 population (1988–91)

USA	22.4
England and Wales	28.7
Germany	21.9
Spain	17.1
Greece	15.2
China	4.6
Japan	6.3
Mexico	8.1
Argentina	20.9

Source: CA: A Cancer Journal for Clinicians, *American Cancer Society*

Lung cancer death rates per 100,000 population (1988–91)

	Men	Women
USA	57.1	24.7
England and Wales	57.0	20.5
Germany	48.7	7.8
Spain	45.2	3.4
Greece	49.8	6.9
China	34.0	14.5
Japan	30.1	8.0
Mexico	16.5	5.9
Argentina	39.2	5.8

Source: CA: A Cancer Journal for Clinicians, *American Cancer Society*

This may not appear to support the argument (certainly the figure for Chinese women is anomalous) – but the Chinese, Japanese and Greeks are ferocious smokers, and a far larger proportion of the male population in these countries smokes than in the US. Yet their death rates are much lower. How can this be? Diet is the obvious answer.

If we compare the top five with the bottom five for all forms of cancer, we get the following:

Men	Women
1 Hungary	Denmark
2 Czechoslovakia	Scotland
3 Uruguay	Hungary
4 Poland	Ireland
5 France	New Zealand
42 Israel	Mexico
43 Venezuela	Greece
44 Mauritius	Japan
45 Ecuador	Puerto Rico
46 Mexico	Mauritius

So, the ingredients for a cancer-free life seem to be: relative poverty, a diet heavy in rice or pasta and vegetables, olive oil or tofu – add in sunshine, music and laughter. The Mediterranean diet of olive oil, pasta, vegetables with a little wine and lots of grapes has been put forward by some as a healthy diet that we should adopt. Certainly it is a tempting one!

A number of people have gone beyond this, and argue on the basis of individual case studies that diets can also *cure* cancer. This view is strongly condemned by the orthodox profession. The authors of *Everyone's Guide to Cancer Therapy* say flatly: 'Following a certain diet or eating certain foods will not make cancer go away. None is known to be helpful. Many result in nutritional deficiencies. Moderation is still the best approach to diet for all medical problems.' But they offer no support for these assertions, which are simply the opinions of surgeons and oncologists with little or no training or experience in the nutritional sciences. The need for evidence and proof cuts both ways. We are free to make up our own minds on the matter. Here, then, are some of the diets for which cancer cures have been claimed.

The five-week juice fast cure
Anne Frahm is one person who believes that diet can cure cancer. Hers was a breast cancer that had metastasised to the backbone – and even to the bone marrow. In her book, *A Cancer Battle Plan*, she describes how for eighteen months she went through every form of conventional therapy – surgery, chemotherapy, radiation, hormone therapy and finally, an autologous bone marrow transplant. They all failed. She refused to 'lie down and play dead', and instead

159

went to see a nutritional counsellor. Following a strict juice diet, she claims that all signs of cancer quickly left her: 'Within five weeks after starting a strict programme of detoxification and diet under the guidance of a nutritional counsellor, my cancer had packed its bags.'

Her recovery was begun by going on a juice fast like this:

8 30 am	Grapefruit juice with olive oil. She brewed a pot of Jason Winter's Tea to sip throughout the day
9 00 am	Apple juice with fibre cleanse, plus enemas
10 00 am	Green drink with vitamin C powder
11 00am	Apple juice with fibre cleanse
Noon	Carrot juice, acidophilus
1 00 pm	Green drink with vitamin C powder
2 00 pm	Apple juice with fibre cleanse
3 00 pm	Carrot juice
4 00 pm	Green drink
5 00 pm	Apple juice with fibre cleanse
6 00 pm	Carrot juice
7 00 pm	Green drink with vitamin C powder
8 00 pm	Carrot juice
9 00 pm	Green drink with vitamin C powder
10 00 pm	Apple juice with fibre cleanse

It is not clear from the book what the green drink consists of. It is either a mixed vegetable juice containing red cabbage, cos lettuce, watercress and green peppers (favoured by proponents of the Gerson diet described below) or it is the barleygreen or wheatgrass drink (also described below). Acidophilus are so-called 'friendly' bacteria that aid digestion and the absorption of nutrients. Jason Winter's Tea is made from chaparral, an American herb.

The ingredients for the juices were organically grown apples and carrots, mixed half-and-half with distilled water. No tap water was allowed. The juices have to be drunk soon after they are made, as the nutrients quickly oxidise.

For Anne Frahm, this was the start of a programme that led on to a largely raw vegetarian diet supported by enzymes, amino acids and vitamin and mineral supplements; strengthened through morale-boosting activities and exercise. And, if we believe what she says, by following this diet rigorously all signs of her cancer were gone in five weeks.

THE WATER QUESTION
Many people believe that tap water, chlorinated and/or fluoridated, or heavy in calcium, is extremely unhealthy and interferes with the absorption of nutrients. The preferred option for them is pure, distilled water. However, critics maintain that distilled water leaches minerals from the system and therefore, in theory, leads to mineral deficiencies. The answer is that, yes, distilled water does leach out minerals, but these are not the organic minerals that the body can use – they are therefore potentially toxic and distilled water is doing the body a favour by removing them.

Others take a different tack, believing that filtered tap water is fine, because the toxic chemicals have been removed. Still others say that filtered tap water is a potential health hazard if the filter is not regularly changed, because the filter becomes loaded with toxins; these eventually leak through, creating water with a very high and very toxic chemical content, instead of providing chemical-free water. This argument goes round and round. Each person has to make his/her own decision. With respect to the juice diet, it seems to me sensible to use bottled, distilled water if this is cheaply and widely available.

THE CASE AGAINST MEAT
Anne Frahm was forbidden by her nutritionist from taking in any animal product, the reason being that they store pollutants from the environment. Dairy products have a 250 per cent higher concentration of pollution – pesticides, etc. – than green leaf vegetables, and 1,500 per cent more than root vegetables. The figures for meat, fish and poultry are double again. Meat also contains all the hormones, antibiotics and other chemicals that are part of modern animal farming. According to T. Colin Campbell, professor of nutritional bio-chemistry at Cornell University: 'Excessive animal protein is at the core of many chronic diseases.'

Animal fats also increase the number of anaerobic bacteria in the human gut; these bacteria create an environment that favours the development of cancer. Anaerobic bacteria live not by oxygen, but by fermentation – and so do cancer cells. In fact, it appears there is a strong case to be made that cancer cells develop as a response to a low oxygen environment. A diet high in animal fats is likely to be low in fibre, so these bacteria stay for longer than they should in the intestine.

So meat is out.

THE PRINCIPLES OF DETOXIFICATION
Alongside her dietary changes, Anne Frahm had a daily enema. The purpose of this procedure is to flush out the colon and so help the regeneration of the liver. Now, the place of the liver in the scheme of things is another focus of dissent. Orthodox surgeons pour scorn on the idea that a poorly functioning liver has anything to do with the development of cancer, but most complementary health practitioners disagree. So do some orthodox doctors. Dr Harold Manner has no doubt that liver dysfunction is the root of the problem: 'The livers of cancer patients have become clogged with many of the poisons they were meant to eliminate. Cancer can be reversed and controlled only if we regenerate the liver. Fortunately for us, the liver is the one organ in the body capable of regenerating itself.'

So purification of the liver is the first step to a cancer-free existence. What causes the liver to become toxic and so dysfunction? Poor elimination of waste in the colon is the answer. Poisonous materials are trapped in the large intestine, and re-absorbed into the bloodstream, where they again go through an increasingly weakened liver. As it becomes less and less able to keep up the work of cleaning the blood, the whole body becomes more toxic.

The most famous exponent of colon health was Norman W. Walker. On the first page of his book, *Colon Health: The Key to a Vibrant Life*, he says: 'Few of us realise that failure to effectively eliminate waste products from the body causes so much fermentation and putrefaction in the large intestine, or colon, that the neglected accumulation of such waste can, and frequently does, result in a lingering demise.' Walker's prescription for a healthy life included half-yearly colonics, vitamin C and raw vegetable juices, particularly carrot juice. Since he lived actively to the age of 109, it is hard to argue with him!

An efficient colon will eliminate food sixteen to twenty-four hours after it has been ingested. Very few British intestines work at this rate. According to the Dunn Nutritional Institute at Cambridge, they average sixty hours, and five days is not unusual. Colonic therapist Pauline Noakes, quoted in *Positive Health* magazine for April/May 1995, says: 'Many people don't realise they are carrying around impacted faecal matter in their colons and that their lack of energy, their irritability, their aches and pains and various ailments are due to the toxic waste in the bowel.'

There is evidence to support this view. Two doctors from the University of California, Nicholas Petrakis and Eileen King, writing in *The Lancet* in 1982, reported that they had studied the breast fluids of 5,000 women. Women who had two or fewer bowel movements per week had four times greater a risk of breast disease (benign or malignant) than those who had one or more bowel movements per day. They also found that the bowels of meat eaters contained greater amounts of mutagenic (potentially harmful) substances than did those of vegetarians.

COLON CLEANSING
Enemas can be undertaken at home with an enema kit bought at a pharmacy. Easier and more effective is to go to a colonic cleansing clinic, but make sure the person giving the therapy is a registered colonic therapist.[14]

And how do you feel after a colonic? Carol Signorella, writing in *Cosmopolitan* magazine in October 1979, said: 'After a year of colonics, my appearance and energy levels were both radically improved. No more draggy mornings or late afternoon slumps. I seem to think more clearly now and I need less sleep. In a word, my body and mind feel marvellously clean.'

Would laxatives work just as well? The answer is a definite no. Colonics clean out the large intestine, but laxatives interfere with the small intestine, which is where digestion and absorption of nutrients occur. Laxatives are also in a sense addictive – for them to continue to be effective, you need to take larger and larger doses.

A word of caution: colon hydrotherapy is not suitable for people with the following conditions: severe cardiac disease, aneurysm, severe anaemia, severe haemorrhoids, cirrhosis, carcinoma of the colon, fistulas, advanced pregnancy, kidney problems and hernia.

There are perfectly good alternatives to a full colonic, one being to take a colonic cleansing treatment. A suspension of Bentonite mud and dried psyllium husks does a good job of taking waste material out of the digestive system. All pharmacies and health shops should be able to offer advice in this area.

Anne Frahm's story is enlightening. Hers is a story where food alone cured cancer, in someone still prepared to fight despite gloomy medical predictions. And she is not alone. In fact, the principle that underlies Frahm's cure has been known for thousands of years. The ancient Hippocratic Oath contains the following, much ignored, statement: 'I will apply dietetic measures for the benefit of the sick according to my ability and judgement.'

The Gerson diet

Max Gerson was an eminent Jewish doctor who fled Nazi Germany for the US – only to find himself persecuted there for his methods of treating cancer. He cured Albert Schweitzer's wife of tuberculosis by dietary means, and on his death in 1959 Schweitzer said of Gerson: 'I see in him one of the most eminent geniuses in the history of medicine.'

The diet Anne Frahm followed was essentially that recommended by Max Gerson in his book *A Cancer Therapy*. This was a summary of thirty years of cancer work using dietary means. Gerson's diet consists of fresh juices of fruits, leaves and vegetables; large quantities of raw fruit and vegetables; vegetables stewed in their own juice, compotes, stewed fruit, potatoes, oatmeal and saltless rye bread.

Everything must be prepared fresh, and salt completely excluded. After six to twelve weeks, animal proteins can be added in the form of pot cheese (saltless and creamless), yoghurt made from skimmed milk, and buttermilk. One underlying principle is to exclude sodium as far as possible and to enrich the body's tissues with potassium – 'to the highest possible degree'. Because it is easier to digest than a normal diet, the body digests each meal faster so larger portions and more frequent meals need to be eaten. Patients are encouraged to eat and drink as much as possible.

The following are forbidden on Gerson's diet: tobacco, salt, spices, tea, coffee, cocoa, chocolate, alcohol, refined sugar, refined flour, candies, ice cream, cream, cake, nuts, mushrooms, soy beans and soy products, pickles, cucumbers, pineapples, all berries (except redcurrants), water (stomach capacity is needed for the juices), avocados, all canned foods, preserves, sulphured peas, lentils and beans, frozen foods, smoked or salted vegetables, dehydrated or powdered foods, bottled juices, and all fats and oils. Hair dyes are also forbidden.

Some items are forbidden at the beginning, but may be introduced to the diet later. These include milk, cheese, butter, fish, meat and eggs. When cooking, aluminium pots must not be used – only stainless steel, glass, enamelware or earthenware.

Although this diet may seem easy to follow in principle, almost everyone on it will suffer some degree of nausea, headaches, gas, depression and even vomiting. Gerson recommends peppermint tea, served with some brown sugar and a piece of lemon, as a cleansing drink to take away any bad tastes or inability to stomach the diet.

Patients also have to expect flare-ups – a sudden incidence of unpleasant symptoms – which do not last more than a few days. These are in fact essential to good health, as they indicate that the body is expelling toxins. Without them, Gerson believes that the patient will not be cured. To ensure that the patient is not damaged by the flare-ups, the body must be detoxified with the use of coffee enemas. It has been argued that it would be very dangerous to combine the Gerson diet with any other effective regime – such as laetrile injections for example – as this might bring on an unexpectedly quick flare-up of dangerous intensity.

Beata Bishop, in her book *My Triumph Over Cancer,* describes how she was cured of her melanoma, which had spread to the groin and which would normally have been fatal within six to eight months, by strictly following the Gerson regime. In her case it took about eighteen months before she was certain she had beaten the disease.

SUPPLEMENTS
Gerson was in favour of lugol solution (half strength) to provide potassium and iodine. 'High potassium/low sodium environments can partially return damaged cell proteins to their normal undamaged configuration,' he wrote.

Potassium deficiency has been shown by others to be present in the following diseases: cancer, leukaemia, diabetes, glaucoma, chronic arthritis, acute and chronic asthma and sinusitis.

Gerson also recommended niacin – 50 mg six times daily, for six months. As for vitamin B12, he was undecided, but he was against the administration of other vitamins because he noticed they sometimes had the effect of causing a tumour to grow back. This is because, he says, non-cancerous tissue in a cancer patient does not react in the same way as normal healthy tissue. That is to say, vitamins may normally be very healthy – but they can have negative effects in people with cancer.

GERSON'S EVIDENCE FOR SUCCESS

In his book, *A Cancer Therapy*, Gerson provides case histories of fifty patients that he cured. One of these was a Mrs E.B., aged forty-eight, married with two children. She presented with a cervical carcinoma which was showing signs of invading neighbouring tissues. The biopsy showed clear malignancy. By the time she reached Gerson, she had already had radiation treatment, but the tumours had returned. He started her on the diet and she kept to it faithfully for eighteen months. At the end, she had no sign of cancer. She slowly weaned herself off the diet, and eleven years later was still cancer-free.

The Gerson Institute claims a success rate of fifty to eighty per cent, depending on the stage of cancer on a person's arrival at the clinic. Other, not necessarily unfriendly, observers estimate a much lower success rate. The Gersons take their readings when the patient goes out by the front door. The observers look at results five years down the road. There may be a simple explanation: the Gerson diet is rigorous, and at home it is easy to slip. Certainly, observers of patients at the clinic are impressed with patients' general level of well-being.[15]

The Moerman diet

In 1938, Dr Cornelis Moerman developed a diet that he used to treat cancer patients who went to see him. He was ridiculed for decades, but in 1987, the Dutch Ministry of Health publicly recognised the Moerman therapy as an effective cancer treatment. Moerman, like many others favouring nutritional health, lived rather longer than many of his orthodox colleagues, dying at ninety-five in 1988.

Moerman began his treatment when a man called Leendert Brinkman went to him seeking help. He had a stomach tumour that had spread to his groin and legs. The doctors had given up on him. Moerman told him to eat as many oranges and lemons as he could. He ate them 'by the truckload until I was up to my eyes in vitamin C'. A year later, he was free of tumours. He went on to live to a healthy old age himself, dying at the age of ninety.

This success led Moerman to develop his nutritional ideas, which he tested on pigeons. Eventually, he came to believe that there were eight substances of vital importance to ideal health, which should be taken in supplemental form as well as through diet. The required daily doses of the eight substances were as follows:

Substance	Dose
Vitamin A	50,000 iu–100,000 iu
B complex vitamins	2 large dose tablets
Vitamin C	as much as can be tolerated
Vitamin E	400–2,200 iu
Citric acid	3 tablespoons of solution: 10–15 g acidum citricum in 300 g water
Iodine	3 tablespoons of solution: iodine spirit (3 per cent), 1–3 drops in 300 g water
Iron	3 teaspoons of solution: undiluted sacharatis ferrici aromatic triplex
Sulfur	1,000 mg

Citric acid helps the blood flow, iodine is important for stimulating the thyroid gland. It also works with sulphur to help oxygenate cells. Iron is needed to prevent anaemia. It should be noted that Moerman's liking for iron is not universally accepted among the vitamin and mineral supplement advocates. Iron has also been implicated, in other studies, as a cancer-promoting agent. It is hard to say at this stage who is right.

Moerman's diet allows a selection of any of the following:

Grains:	whole-grain breads and pastas, brown rice, barley, oat bran, wheat germ, wheat or corn flakes.
Dairy:	butter, buttermilk, cream cheese, cottage cheese, egg yolks, plain live yoghurt.
Vegetables:	most vegetables lightly steamed. Highly recommended: beet juice and carrot juice. Limited intake: brussels sprouts, cauliflower, parsley.
Fruit:	most fruits. Highly recommended: mixed fresh orange and lemon juice.
Others:	bay leaf, garlic, herb tea, nutmeg, cold-pressed olive and sunflower oil.

Prohibited foods are meat, fish and shellfish, alcohol, animal fats, artificial colourings, beans, peas, lentils, mushrooms, potatoes, red cabbage, sauerkraut, cheeses with high fat and salt content, margarine and other hydrogenated oils, coffee, cocoa or caffeine-containing teas, egg whites, sugar, salt, white flour and tobacco.

MOERMAN'S EVIDENCE FOR SUCCESS

As we can see, there is a great deal of overlap with the Gerson diet. Of the two, Gerson's is clearly more rigorous, in that it stresses that the intake must be raw – but if even Dr Moerman's lighter regime is considered effective, then some leeway is clearly permitted. But is there any proof that it is effective? A number of doctors interested in Moerman's diet set up a research project which followed 150 patients. The results should be compared with the figure of cancer patients cured by orthodox means, which is approximately forty per cent overall.

Solid tumour cancer patients

Number cured with Moerman therapy alone:	60 (40%)
Number cured with Moerman therapy after other treatment:	55 (36.66%)
Total cured with Moerman therapy:	115 (76.66%)
Number who were not cured:	35 (23.33%)
Total number in study:	150 (99.99%)

Source: 1983 SIKON Study Data (adapted from Ruth Jochems, 1990)

Results of small studies like this are open to many objections, but the results certainly indicate that further research should be done. Unlike the Dutch Ministry of Health, the American Cancer Society does not accept that the Moerman diet is an effective cancer treatment.

The macrobiotic diet

Modern macrobiotics was developed in Japan at the turn of the century. Two educators, Dr Sagen Ishitsuka and Yukikazu Sakurazawa, cured themselves of serious chronic illnesses by changing their diets to one consisting of brown rice, miso soup, sea vegetables and other traditional foods. Sakurazawa went to Paris in the 1920s and – using the name George Ohsawa – began to spread the word.

Ohsawa's macrobiotic diet is based on Eastern philosophy and takes its starting point with yin (the dark, passive, female) and yang (the light, active, male forces), which must be maintained in a state of harmony. The body, as with everything else in the universe, must maintain a healthy balance between these two forces. As each person is unique, the point of balance is different for every individual. Cancer tumours also have yin and yang characteristics. For example, while cancer of the tongue is yang, all other tumours of the upper digestive tract are considered to be yin.

From a macrobiotic point of view, cancer is simply a sign, among others, that the body is in a disharmonious state. The objective, then, is to restore harmony. The only way we can achieve this is through dietary means, such as that recommended by Michio Kushi and Alex Jack, in their book *The Cancer-Prevention Diet*. This is true even when there appears to be a direct carcinogenic cause – e.g. a skin cancer caused by too much exposure to sunlight. They explain this in the following way. People in the West eat a lot of sugars, fats, dairy products and canned foods and drinks. These create an acidic state, which is yin. When exposed to the sun, a strong yang factor, the yin items rise to the surface and a tumour results. People in tropical countries whose diets consist of grains, tubers, seeds, vegetables and locally grown fruit with only a small amount of animal food will not get skin cancer, no matter how long they are out in the sun, because their blood and tissues do not contain these yin toxins. Certainly, inhabitants of hot countries do not appear to suffer higher incidences of melanoma.

The macrobiotic diet consists of the following.

Food Item	Percentage Daily Intake	Form
Whole grains	50–60	Should be eaten in whole form, not cracked. Brown rice should be pressure cooked, not boiled. Breads should not contain yeast; chapatis, tortillas and sourdough bread are recommended.
Soup	5–10	One or two bowls of miso or tamari soup. Miso is a kind of fermented soybean paste. Miso should have aged more than twelve years, and be made of organically grown soy beans.*
Vegetables	25–30	Should be fresh. Up to a third can be eaten raw.
Beans and sea vegetables	5–10	
Oils		Unrefined sesame, corn or mustard seed oils. Unrefined safflower, sunflower, soy and olive oils can be used occasionally.
Others		Sea salt – though meals should be neither too salty nor too bland. Salt should be used in the cooking, not at the table.

* It is known that miso contains a number of anti-angiogenesis substances that interfere with tumour growth.

The way in which we eat food is also important. Each mouthful should be chewed fifty to seventy times before swallowing. Avoid eating three hours before sleeping. Eat only when hungry; drink only when thirsty. Give thanks and respect to the whole world of living beings, and to all those who made the food available.

One of the surprising features of the macrobiotic diet is its avoidance of fruits. This avoidance isn't absolute, but fruits are advised only occasionally, in the proper climatic zone and in the appropriate season. A person in Europe in winter should not be eating bananas or oranges. Also to be avoided, in addition to red meats, dairy products and any form of processed food, are cooking spices and herbs, butter or margarine, iodised salt, ginseng, eggs and yoghurt. Another surprise is the ban on any kind of vitamin or mineral supplement.

EVIDENCE FOR THE MACROBIOTIC DIET'S SUCCESS

Kushi and Jack offer a number of stories of people being cured. One was Jean Kohler, a fifty-six-year-old pianist and professor of music. One summer, he suddenly became aware of an itch that spread up his leg. After several tests, doctors discovered a massive tumour on his pancreas. Pancreatic tumours are almost always fatal. He was told nothing could be done and that he had anywhere from one month to three years to live. He accepted chemotherapy, but after a few days decided that he didn't want to continue with such debilitating treatment. Kohler started to look for an alternative therapy, and was referred to the Kushi Institute in Boston. He started a macrobiotic regime and within six months all signs of cancerous activity had ceased. This was confirmed by medical tests.

Kohler lived another seven years and then died of something else entirely. He publicised his case whenever he could, and even wrote a book about it. Kushi and Jack quote him as saying: 'The best thing to ever happen to me was having so-called terminal cancer.'

In another case, Dr Vivien Newbold, an emergency care doctor in Philadelphia, became interested in macrobiotics when her husband had a metastatic cancer of the colon. He reduced the cancer by seventy per cent by going on a

171

macrobiotic diet. Dr Newbold subsequently wrote an article detailing the effect of a macrobiotic diet on six cases; the five cases who stuck with the diet went into total remission for over five years. This article was rejected by three professional magazines, and Newbold was told by the American Cancer Society that it was 'of no interest to us'.

In 1993, however, the *Journal of the American College of Nutrition* published a study of the effects of the macrobiotic diet on people with pancreatic cancer. After one year, fifty-two per cent of those on the diet were still alive, compared with only ten per cent of the controls – a 500 per cent increase in one-year survival rates.

Kushi regrets that too often people only start to look at macrobiotics when other attempts have failed: 'Only about fifteen to twenty per cent among my visitors are able to get better. If they would come to see me at an earlier stage of illness, or had greater family support, the percentage would be much higher.'[16]

The Bristol detox diet

This is mainly a juice diet, which is completely vegan. It consists of ninety per cent raw food and is strictly salt and sugar free – not even honey should be taken. Each meal can be accompanied by wholemeal bread or wholegrain rice.

The foods that should be eaten may be chosen from the following list:

Eat plenty of: alfalfa sprouts, almonds, beansprouts, sprouted aduki and mung beans, runner beans, soy beans, beetroot, broccoli, Brussels sprouts, carrot juice, cauliflower, chicory, fennel, fenugreek, kale, kohlrabi, leeks, summer lettuce, home-made muesli, rolled oats, brown rice, rye bread, sprouted sunflower seeds, wheat berries.

Eat in moderation: apple, apricot kernels, apricots, artichokes, bananas, bay leaves, beans of all kinds, wholemeal bread, bulgar wheat, carrots, cashews, Chinese cabbage, corn on the cob, courgettes, couscous, fresh figs, grapefruit, grapes, hazelnuts, kiwi fruit, lentils, marrow, melon, millet, fresh dried mint, oranges, peas, sweet potatoes, pumpkin, wholewheat semolina, spinach, swedes, turnip.

The only surprise in this list is the low value given to the onion family, especially to garlic. As with the macrobiotic diet, great attention should be given to chewing the food slowly, in a calm frame of mind.

For further information contact the Bristol Cancer Help Centre.[17]

Fasting

Doctors, by and large, take it as an article of faith that it is important to eat well in order to maintain the health and vigour of the body. Even Max Gerson opposed the idea of fasting, because it would result in vitamin and mineral deficiencies, so weakening the body further. However, there is a great deal of evidence that fasting can have a positive effect on health.

The masterwork on fasting is Herbert Shelton's *The Science and Fine Art of Fasting*, which was first published in 1934. In a foreword to this edition, Shelton describes the case of Dr Henry Tanner, who, in 1877, felt he could no longer cope with the pains and illnesses that were plaguing him. It was an accepted fact at that time that to go without food for ten days was a certain way to enter the beyond. So Tanner, preferring to ease his way to the next world rather than to commit an act of violence against his person, took to his bed and refused all food. So far from dying, he found that, by the forty-second day, he had recovered. When he announced this to his colleagues, he was denounced as a fraud. To prove he was not, he undertook another forty-two-day fast, under the supervision of the United States Medical College of New York. He was placed in a fenced-off area and a watch was kept on him by sixty volunteer physicians.

Shelton argues that fasting, far from being an abnormal reaction to ill-health, is actually a very natural one. He points to the fact that wounded or ill animals often refuse food until they are on the mend. When we are ill, we often have no appetite for food. The clear implication is that the body does not wish to have food – and since the body is credited with healing powers, what it wants is probably good for it. Bear in mind that some animals go for months in hibernation without any food or drink.

Fasting as a way of achieving physical and spiritual

purification is a common aspect of religious life – it is frequently mentioned in the Bible. The ancient Greek philosophers were also frequent fasters. Before someone could be accepted as a student by Pythagoras, he had to undergo a forty-day fast. In addition to its therapeutic value it was, presumably, a means of determining who had the necessary discipline for study. Asclepius is the Greek god of healing, and healing through fasting was a regular feature of life at his temples. Many of the great ancient doctors, from Hippocrates to Avicenna, have recommended healing fasts.

Fasting works because of a process known as autolysis, or self-digestion. For example, when a tadpole starts to turn into a frog, it first grows four legs. It then rids itself of its tail – but the tail does not fall off. Instead, it is taken back into the body and absorbed. While this is occurring, the tadpole-frog does not eat. Autolysis is a controlled process, by which the least essential parts of the body are self-digested. This is also true in starvation; the body seeks to preserve the most essential organs and tissues by allowing the least important to be digested first. This is very important when it comes to cancer. Cancer tumours are recognised as being the least essential tissues in the body, and so are easy victims of the autolytic process.

HOW TO FAST

Is fasting hard to do? Apparently not. After a few days, it seems that the hunger goes. Many fasters experience clear improvements in their mental abilities. Shelton says: 'All of man's intellectual and emotional qualities are given new life.' The first week of a fast should be done during a period of rest, where no physical demands are made on the faster. But after that, it appears, there is no problem accomplishing quite demanding tasks. However, Shelton's view on this subject is pithy: 'On general principles, working during a long fast is to be severely condemned. It has been done. It can often be done. But it should not be done.'

Water should not be drunk in large quantities; instead, the faster should drink when thirsty. Shelton is also opposed to the use of enemas, believing that they retard the process of healing. This is a matter on which there is much disagreement – the present European practice strongly encourages the taking of enemas to rid the body of any toxic build-up.

EVIDENCE FOR THE SUCCESS OF FASTING

Shelton gives a number of examples of people who were cured of cancer by means of a fast, but he cautions that there is a wide variation in response from person to person. In some people, the tumour will be devoured quickly, in others slowly. In one case, a cancer cure required a fast of twenty-one days followed shortly after by another of seventeen days. This was considered by Shelton to be abnormally long. Another woman had a speedier response: '[After] exactly three days without food, the "cancer" and all its attendant pain were gone. There had been no recurrence after thirteen years, and I think that we are justified in considering the condition remedied.'

Shelton does accept that, when a cancer tumour has grown very large, it may take years of on-and-off fasting to absorb it – and even then it may not be possible. But on the whole, he is extremely optimistic about the cancer-curing potential of a fast.

Dr Virginia Vertrano, who took over Shelton's clinic, reported: 'I kept a lady alive for ten years longer than the doctors said she'd live, by fasting her once a year and keeping her on an all raw-food diet between the fasts. She had a very malignant breast tumour.' (Quoted by Richard Walters, 1993) However, Vertrano cautions that some tumours return once the fast has finished.

Is there any more recent evidence that fasting works? Certainly there is evidence that low-calorie diets are health promoting, as the following examples show. In 1942, Albert Tannenbaum, cancer researcher at Michael Reese Hospital in Chicago, found that mice on a low-calorie diet had substantially lower incidences of induced breast tumours, lung tumours and sarcoma than mice on an unrestricted diet. He also found that mice on a high-fat diet had a significantly higher incidence of spontaneous breast cancer. Tumours also appeared much earlier in mice fed with a high-fat diet.

In 1944, cancer researcher J. Saxton reported that a special strain of laboratory mice with a high leukaemia rate, and fed only forty per cent of a normal diet, reduced their leukaemia incidence from sixty-five to ten per cent. A 1947 study found that the opposite effect also occurred. A high-protein diet increased leukaemia incidence. A 1982 study at UCLA found that mice fed twenty-eight to forty-three per cent fewer calories lived ten to twenty per cent longer than their controls, and had fewer tumours of the lymphatic system

Fasting has a major theoretical defect as a cancer treatment, in that the original imbalance of vitamins, minerals and/or essential fatty acids that may have helped to give rise to the cancer in the first place is not rectified. It seems sensible then, if a fast appears to be an attractive way of dealing with a cancer, to fortify the body with high levels of the relevant supplements before and after the fast. Also, at the end of the fast, you should not go for a sudden blow-out. A juice diet should be the first step on the road to resuming a normal diet, with some thin oatmeal porridge or vegetable soup working slowly up to a vegetable stew.

The grape diet
The grape cure is not the first, or only, single food diet that has been put forward as a health cure. In Victorian times, a diet of pure raw lean beef was considered to be the perfect health regime. Similarly, in India, a diet of urine alone for several weeks on end is supposed to be cleansing. A diet of plain steamed brown rice has also been proposed by some as a cleansing diet that releases a great deal of healing energy.

The grape cure consists of eating grapes – skin, pips and all – and nothing but grapes, for a period of four weeks. This grape cure is probably an ancient Mediterranean folk cure. Basil Shackleton was a very ill man when he came, almost at the end of his tether, to the grape diet. His only remaining kidney was diseased and would not respond to drugs. He had been chronically ill for over forty years, having caught bilharzia when a young boy growing up in Africa. In despair, he turned to a cure that he had only vaguely heard about – a diet of grapes. In his book, *The Grape Cure*, he explain what happened: 'There is magic in the world – and there are miracles! After twenty-three days on the treatment, I came through, looking and feeling twenty years younger – and I was completely and perma-

176

nently cured! My body became charged with a new vitality. I felt radiant and whole.'

The grape cure Shackleton recommends consists simply of eating as many grapes as desired – no drugs, no other foods, no liquids other than hot or cold water (hot for those times when you will feel nauseated). Water may be drunk at all times, but not within an hour after eating the grapes as this will only dilute the strength of the natural chemicals in the fruit. The grapes must be washed thoroughly – and soaked two or three times – to remove any pesticides on the skin.

During this cure, there must be at least one bowel movement every two days – if not, an enema or colonic is necessary – because the faeces are the main channel for the elimination of toxic matter. Shackleton also recommends a glycerin suppository for the purpose of encouraging a bowel movement.

Anyone following a toxin-removing regime will suffer badly in the first week from headaches, but these will gradually disappear. These headaches are a barometer of your condition. The worse they are, the more toxins you have in your body that need to be eliminated.

Juice fasts

Austrian herbalist, Rudolf Breuss, claims that a fast in which the faster drinks only 500 ml (18 fl oz) a day of his special juice is an effective cancer treatment. His juice should be made from the following vegetables in approximately these proportions: beet (300 g/11 oz), carrot (100 g/3½ oz), celery (100 g/3½ oz), a radish (50 g/1¾ oz) and a small potato. Press these vegetables through a tea sieve and drink the juice, but don't eat the remaining solid sediment. Instead of using potato in this way, you can make a tea of potato peel. Cook a handful of peel with two cups of water, simmering for two to four minutes. If the resulting liquid tastes unpleasant, don't drink it. Taste is an indication of the body's desire to take in a particular food.

This juice should be supplemented with sage tea. According to Breuss, sage tea drunk every day will keep you free of almost all illness. It is made by putting two teaspoons of fresh sage in 500 ml (18 fl oz) boiling water. This should be boiled for three minutes, left to steep for ten minutes, and then drunk.

Individual foods as medicines

BARLEY GREEN ESSENCE AND WHEATGRASS

Barley Green Essence is the concentrated extract of young barley, rye and oat shoots which have been allowed to grow until the leaves have become dark green. This was developed by a Japanese scientist, Yoshide Hagiwara, to support his own health. Hagiwara believes that: 'The leaves of the cereal grasses provide the nearest thing this planet offers to the perfect food.'

Barley Green Essence is available as a powder and in capsule forms, though Hagiwara personally recommends the powder form. The potassium content of this product is very high, which makes it a good food for people under high stress, when blood potassium levels will show a marked tendency to fall. Potassium is therefore being used up at a high rate, and needs to be replaced. If it is not, then the result is fatigue.

Barley Green Essence is also very high in vitamins. It has six times as much beta-carotene and three times as much vitamin C as spinach. It is high in folic acid and nicotinic acid (important B vitamins) as well as biotin, chlorophyll and choline. Chlorophyll, which in plants is the substance that transforms the sun's light into food, is very close in chemical structure to the haemoglobin in our blood – the only difference being one of its mineral components. Blood is bonded with iron, while chlorophyll is bonded by magnesium. Hagiwara believes that the blood can be reinvigorated by eating chlorophyll.

Wheatgrass drinks were common in Europe during the 1920s, and from there Ann Wigmore brought them to the US. Both Hagiwara and Wigmore consider their products to be effective components of a holistic, anti-cancer dietary regime. There are now a number of similar products on the market, containing additional herbs, enzymes, and so on.

Wheatgrass contains over one hundred nutrients. It is the anchor around which Ann Wigmore has developed her Wheatgrass Therapy. The other components are the eating of raw foods – especially sprouting beans – meditation and detoxification.[18]

LINSEED OIL AND COTTAGE CHEESE

The importance of linseed oil in the fight against cancer was first proposed by an eminent German bio-chemist, Dr Johanna Budwig. She meticulously analysed thousands of blood samples from people who were ill, and compared these samples with others taken from people who were well. She discovered that those who were seriously ill (with cancer, diabetes and other ailments) were, without exception, deficient in linoleic acid. They were also deficient in phosphatides, which are required for normal cell division, and albumin – a blood producing lipoprotein, itself a combination of linoleic acid and proteins.

Without linoleic acid, the body can't produce haemoglobin, and without haemoglobin, the body can't carry vital oxygen to the tissues. This then creates a low oxygen environment, ideal for the development of cancer. The cancer patient becomes more anaemic and the inevitable result is death. Without the phosphatides to stabilise cell growth, cancer tumours grow uncontrollably. Without the albumin, the haemoglobin changes from a healthy red to a diseased yellow-green colour, and cannot do its job of circulating oxygen around the system. To correct the situation, Dr Budwig surmised, the patient should take in large quantities of linoleic acid and sulphur-based protein.

The source she chose for linoleic acid was pure virgin, cold-pressed, unprocessed linseed oil (also known as flaxseed oil). Flaxseed oil is very high in Omega 3 fatty acids, as is EPA (eicosapentaenoic acid), which is found in fish oils and seaweeds. For sulphur-based proteins, Budwig first chose skim milk, later changing to low-fat cottage cheese. She tested this on cancer patients, giving them 40 grams of linseed oil in 100 grams of skim milk, with 25 grams of whole milk to make the mixture easier to blend. The result was exactly as she had predicted: the cancer tumours receded slowly, and the haemoglobin regained its healthy red colour.

The basic combination can be taken in any quantity – the more the better. Flaxseed oil is sold at most health food shops. It must be kept in dark bottles and in cool places. It quickly loses its potency in light conditions, so it must be made up fresh each time it is eaten. However, citrus fruits prevent it from being effective.

It is recommended that this mixture be supported by a diet that contains fresh fruits, fresh vegetables, unprocessed cereals, fresh cold-water fish, six to eight daily glasses of bottled distilled water, and herbal teas. Foods to avoid include: all processed oils, fried foods, sugar, artificial sweeteners and any processed food containing preservatives or chemical additives.

It is also useful to wrap the affected part with towels soaked in linseed oil (do not warm or heat the oil). Healing aromatherapy oils can be added at the same time.

Support for the success of Omega 3 oil
Support for the oil's anti-cancer effects comes from Barry Sears, author of *The Zone*, a book proposing a radically new way of viewing diet. He lays the cause of both health and disease at the doorstep of a group of chemicals called eicosanoids – there are good eicosanoids and bad eicosanoids. A diet high in total fat consumption (particularly Omega 6 fatty acids) will produce more bad eicosanoids – whereas a diet that has a high Omega 3 oil content favours the production of good eicosanoids.

Sears attributes the success of the macrobiotic diet to the fact that it results in a very good oil intake. Where he faults it is in the fact that it favours high carbohydrate consumption, which again encourages the production of bad eicosanoids. For this reason, Sears also does not approve of strict vegetarian diets for cancer patients.

Sears, a bio-chemist who owns a number of patents on ways of delivering chemotherapy drugs, nevertheless argues that: 'Caloric restriction – coupled with the correct macronutrient composition – is far more effective than any drug in the prevention or treatment of cancer.' For Sears, the best anti-cancer diet:

- is low in calories
- contains no red meats or egg yolk
- is low in total fat, but high in fish oils (especially from salmon)
- has a protein to carbohydrate ratio of 3 grams of protein for 4 grams of carbohydrate, with most carbohydrates coming from fruit or fibre-rich vegetables.

GARLIC
Garlic is a very potent anti-pathogen. Recent tests at the University of Alabama Medical School suggest that it is as

powerful as many modern anti-bacterial and anti-viral drugs, with minimal toxicity – 'the only toxicity is social,' said one commentator wryly. To beat the social side-effects, garlic can be taken in de-odorised pill form. For garlic breath, chew on parsley leaves. In China, garlic extract is used in IV infusions to treat systemic fungal infections. One or two cloves a day can be sure to keep the doctor away! Garlic is also a potentially useful protective agent for the liver, and a very good source of selenium, germanium, amino acids and enzymes.

Garlic can be eaten raw, 25–100 grams (1–3½ oz) a day, or taken in the form of de-odorised pills or liquid extracts. Kyolic® brand garlic pills are highly regarded, because of the attention paid to the soil that the garlic is grown in and the quality of the cold-ageing process that the whole cloves of garlic undergo.

Although garlic is the most potent member of the onion family, the other members are also associated with good health. As well as onion, these include asparagus, chives, leeks and sarsaparilla. A string of garlic was hung up outside the door during times of plague, or around the necks of the ill.

Garlic can be applied externally with good effect. A poultice can be made of finely chopped or juiced garlic, slippery elm, pokeroot – a wild plant common to the southern states of America whose leaves appear in salads – castor oil, vinegar, water and, on open wounds, cayenne pepper. Place this mixture with any additional herbs desired on a gauze pad and apply it to the skin closest to the tumour site. The poultice should be washed off in a shower every twelve hours and the area under the poultice allowed to breathe for one to two hours before a new poultice is applied. The result will burn the skin and may even raise a blister. These burns can be treated with lavender essential oil, aloe vera or comfrey. DMSO (see page 241) can be added to the poultice to aid absorption through the skin. This is claimed to be a very powerful anti-tumour treatment.

CRUCIFEROUS VEGETABLES
This vegetable family, which includes broccoli, cauliflower, cabbage, Brussels sprouts, collards, kale, mustard greens,

turnips and turnip greens, contains a number of compounds that have shown inhibitory action on cancers in animals. Communities that eat higher amounts of these vegetables show reduced incidence of cancer.

SEA VEGETABLES

We call them seaweeds, but the Japanese, in particular, have a liking for the edible plants that grow in the sea. One seaweed extract marketed under the name Viva Natural has been found to be active against lung cancer and leukaemia. There is also some evidence that these vegetables may be active against breast cancer. Kelp and dulce are widely available seaweed extracts. Kombu, however, should be eaten in moderation, as it contains very high iodine levels and can induce temporary hyperthyroidism (this stops when levels of iodine are reduced).

BITTER MELON

This is a light-to-medium green Chinese melon, recognisable for being 10–15 cm (4–6 inches) long, with knobbled ridges – a very bumpy vegetable! Its botanical name is *Momordica charantia*. In Cantonese it is known as fu (bitter) gwa or leung (cooling) gwa. When lightly fried or steamed, it has a sharply tart but not unpleasant taste. It is very popular in the summer months, when it is eaten to cool the body down. This 'cooling' effect may be felt as a cleansing or purifying process. It is not recommended for pregnant women, as it can induce spontaneous abortion.

For cancer patients, it is suggested that the bitter melon fruit and leaves are eaten together in large daily quantities. Bitter melon is being recommended by a number of AIDS activist groups as an immune support for people infected with HIV. For these purposes, the fruit of the bitter melon is not used. A 'tea' is made from 450 grams (1 lb) of leaves and vines and 2 litres (3½ pints) of water, brought to the boil and then simmered for sixty to ninety minutes (stirring every twenty minutes), and then cooled. Alternatively, leaves and water can be put through a blender. In both cases, the resulting liquid is strained to remove solid particles. It is then taken into the body through the colon in the form of a retention enema. This way of taking bitter melon may also be beneficial for cancer patients.

Bitter melon tea appears to be, like garlic, a powerful anti-viral agent, and is also effective against the herpes simplex virus.

Some studies seeking to work with the substance identified as the active agent had to be cancelled, as this substance was found to be highly toxic in its pure form. Bitter melon presents a problem of classification – is it a herb or a food item?

FOODS RICH IN ABSCISIC ACID
Abscisic acid is one of nature's most potent anti-cancer weapons, according to the cancer researcher, Dr Livingston-Wheeler. The foods richest in these substances are carrots, mangoes, grapes, avocados, pears, strawberries, tomatoes, lima beans, seeds, nuts and green leafy and root vegetables.

FOODS RICH IN STARCH
Information on foods rich in starch arose out of an epidemiological study of twelve countries. Those with high average starch intake scored low on cancers of the bowel, colon and rectum. Australian men and American women eat the least starch – 100 grams (3½ oz) or less a day – while the Chinese eat 370 grams (12½ oz) or more. Australian men suffer colon cancer at a rate of 25 per 100,000, while the rate for the Chinese is only 6.3.

The benefit comes from starch that is not digested in the small intestine. This so-called resistant starch is then broken down by bacteria in the large intestine. This produces a short-chain fatty acid called butyrate, which may have the effect of reducing the proliferation of cancer cells. Slightly unripe bananas are good – ripe ones are not, because the resistant starch has been converted to sugars. Another good source of resistant starch is cold boiled potatoes.

Foods to avoid
1. All refined polyunsaturated oils, i.e. cooking oils and margarines. These have a depressing effect on the immune system. They also interfere with the cells' use of oxygen to burn the basic foodstuffs to produce energy. The result is a cell that is potentially cancerous.
2. All animal fats. These should be avoided because they are full of synthetic hormones, antibiotics and pesticides. According to Dr Livingston, chicken especially should be

avoided because it contains, in very high quantities, a microbe implicated in cancer generation, which she called progenitor cryptocides. Since intensively farmed livestock is often fed chicken manure, beef and pork meats may also be affected. This microbe can change its form from something similar to a bacteria to another form similar to a virus. This microbe is present in large numbers in cancer patients. Milk may also be dangerous, according to Dr Livingston, as eighty to ninety per cent of cattle carry leukaemia.

Nutritional therapy – an overview

There is general agreement that seventy to ninety per cent of cancers are caused by lifestyle and environment; of these, at least half are in some way related to diet and nutrition, while a further thirty per cent are the result of cigarette smoking. Some studies supporting a nutritional approach to prevention or cure are summarised below.

A large-scale study in New Zealand in 1994 showed that vegetarians had less than half the cancer risk of their meat-eating friends and neighbours.

A fifty-year study in England and Wales found that breast cancer mortality decreased from the beginning of the Second World War, because intake of animal fats and sugar fell due to rationing. In 1954, consumption of these items returned to pre-war levels. However, breast cancer rates did not return until about 1969, suggesting that there is a fifteen-year time lag between ingestion and development of the disease.

Seventh Day Adventists, of whom roughly half are vegetarian, have significantly lower cancer levels than average – eighty-four per cent less cervical cancer and thirty to forty-four per cent fewer leukaemias.

The Hunza people of northern Pakistan are renowned for their freedom from degenerative diseases. Dr Robert McCarrison, who visited the area from 1904 to 1911, said: 'I never saw a case of cancer.' He attributed their health and longevity to their diet of wholewheat chapatis, barley, maize, green leafy vegetables, beans and apricots. Later, while experimenting on rats, he found that rats fed on the Hunza diet remained healthy and free of disease, while those who ate the normal Indian diet contracted heart disease, cancer and other ailments.

The herbal approach

In an era that prides itself on its science, herbs may seem to represent a throwback to the dark ages, conjuring up images of monks stirring cauldrons or old women plucking grasses from the hedgerow. However, there are very good reasons for taking that prejudice by the scruff of its neck and kicking it out of the house. Herbs are coming back with a vengeance, for very good reasons.

The use of herbal remedies goes back to the beginnings of time, and many animals also make use of the medicinal qualities of herbs. Ethologists know that monkeys eat plants both for the purposes of getting a drug high and recuperating from an illness. Some monkeys know which plants will help them get rid of parasites, others know which ones have a contraceptive effect. This knowledge of herbal medicines among animals, known as zoopharmacognosy, is not restricted to monkeys. One animal researcher once had to pursue a berserk pregnant elephant for twenty miles until she came to a tree and tore it to shreds as she ate the bark. Shortly afterwards, she gave birth to her calf. On analysis, the medicinal qualities of the bark were found to contain a chemical that was helpful in aiding delivery.

The use of plant medicines by animals poses a problem for those who believe that knowledge advances only through scientific research. Have the monkeys been scientific? What, then, of the elephant? It has, in fact, been suggested that all animals, including humans, have an instinct for recognising what is good and what is not good to eat – and for knowing which plants may be good for specific ailments. This instinct will express itself in intuitions, vague feelings and even dreams – all very unscientific. But if we do have such instincts – more refined or accessible in some individuals than others – then the implications are enormous.

The medicinal properties of many plants have been known to man, too, for centuries. Hippocrates used to prescribe willow bark for a number of ailments – long after his time, the active ingredient was isolated and marketed as aspirin. With the rise of science, single substance drugs became the order of the day, and herbalism to a large extent went underground. It became a woman's area of expertise, where recipes were handed on from mother to daughter.

In eighteenth-century North America, a woman by the name of Mary Johnson came to the attention of the medical authorities. It appeared she was working as a healer and was claiming success in the treatment of cancer. The House of Burgesses of the General Assembly of Virginia appointed a committee to look into the case. Mary Johnson's medicine was a mixture of garden sorrel, celandine, persimmon bark and spring water. The committee took evidence over a period of six or seven years, 1748–54. They listened to the testimony of many witnesses who had taken the remedy and been cured. The result? Mrs Johnson was awarded £100 to aid her work.

Chemicals and herbs – a fundamental difference

The above is a rare tale of diligent and generous assessment. The outcome of the investigation would be very different today – for the simple fact is, herbs represent a fundamental challenge to the ruling medical paradigm. This paradigm argues as follows: if there is anecdotal evidence that a herb has a specific medicinal property, then the plant in question may contain a specific chemical which can be called the active ingredient. The plant is then studied to determine what its chemical contents are, and these are tested one at a time until the active ingredient is identified. Then this isolated substance can be tested scientifically to assess its range of action and ideal dosage. It will also, incidentally, be possible to manufacture the chemical directly in large quantities without having to go through the arduous and expensive process of extraction from plant sources.

This illustrates the fact that the ultimate aim of chemical research is to create on an industrial scale single chemicals in pure form. By contrast, Mary Johnson proceeded by mixing a number of herbs together – in what proportions is not known. She was operating according to very different principles. While the scientist is looking for pure unadulterated chemicals, the herbalist is seeking to blend combinations of many different chemicals. There is good evidence that Mrs Johnson's approach is the way forward. We can see this easily with two simple and common examples. Smokers take into their bodies a great deal of nicotine every time they light up a cigarette. Yet, if they were to place one drop of pure unadulterated nicotine on their skin, they would have only seconds to live: pure nicotine is one of the most potent poisons known to man.

Marijuana, to take another example, has clearly demonstrated medicinal qualities. It is known to help relieve eye pressure in the case of glaucoma and to reduce the effects of nausea – making it a very suitable herbal supplement for people undergoing chemotherapy. Unfortunately, its status as an illegal drug makes it difficult for a herbalist to prescribe. Scientists therefore proceeded to isolate from the marijuana plant an active ingredient, which they called THC. This was approved as a drug in 1985. The result? *Science News* reported that: 'Many patients and physicians claim that purified THC is not nearly as effective as a puff of pot'; commenting on its side-effects, one writer noted that 'Fifty per cent of the patients said they'd rather throw up' than take THC.

There is no evidence that single substance chemicals are superior to herbs. In fact, there is good reason to believe they may be inferior. Why? For three reasons.

Firstly, there is the problem of resistance. Invading organisms, such as bacteria and viruses, are able to resist pure chemical forms quite effectively. That is why bacteria are increasingly becoming resistant to antibiotics, and also why the body is able to resist chemotherapeutic drugs. Remember that doctors are now *mixing* these chemotherapeutic agents; that is, they are starting to mimic the herbalist.

Secondly, the negative side-effects of purified molecular forms – the basis of all drugs – are rarely present when herbs are used. This is not to say that herbs are always safe, for they are not. But such side-effects as there are tend to be muffled by the presence of the surrounding chemicals in the composite herbal structures found in nature.

The third, and perhaps the most important, reason is the

fact that the concept of the single active ingredient is almost certainly wrong. It is much more likely, in any herbal substance, that one dominant active chemical is boosted by the presence of others. When separated from these surrounding molecules, it may no longer have the desired effect. The process by which two chemicals contribute to a more pronounced effect is known as synergy. It may even be possible that none of the ingredients of a particular plant have any effect on their own, but when present in an organic whole, they combine to have an effect.

This point about 'organic wholes' is central to the herbalist's credo. In the herb, compounds are interconnected in a coherent structure and have certain qualities both separately and together that are entirely absent from all artificially created chemicals. As we have seen, organic germanium is health giving, while chemically identical, inorganic germanium causes kidney damage. If we follow this argument, then we needn't be too despondent at the banning of laetrile and germanium – they are present in abundant quantities in dietary form, a form which is likely to be more effective.

Some people illustrate the difference between organic and inorganic forms by using the metaphor of music. If you press the A key on a piano, you will create three kinds of vibrations. One is the vibration that creates the note A, but mixed with this will be overtones that make it clear to any listener that the note A comes from a piano and not a violin or clarinet. In addition, there will be other vibrations that stem from the interaction of the particular musician and the particular instrument. The writer Dean Black, in describing this fact, makes the point that if the music were a herb, then the active element would be the A note – it is the most noticeable property of the sound, and the only one that can stand alone: '[However] None of the three vibrations define the note's entire function, and some of the note's most interesting properties – its "piano-ness" and its "tone quality" – don't exist anywhere except as they somehow emerge like magic when the vibrations blend together.' (Black, 1988) Herbalists believe that the chemical properties of a whole plant operate in the same way, and that we lose these properties when we break the plant up.

Not everyone is convinced by this argument. They maintain that drugs are better than herbs, because herbs contain too many ingredients in variable concentrations. One ounce (or 25 g) of ma-huang grown in the US may be very different in quality from the same weight of the same herb grown in China. There is no standardisation, so it is impossible adequately to test the precise effects of any herb. Because these objections don't apply to drugs, they say, drugs must be better. But no logic forces us to accept that just because a drug is easier to experiment with in a laboratory it is therefore a better form of medicine.

The conflict of herb versus drug is, in miniature, the war between factory and nature, between West and East, between 'scientific' techno-medicine and holistic healing. How is it that there is no official recognition that herbs play a part in the treatment of cancer? Because it is impossible to prove this effect under the conditions of proof currently laid down – and it would cost millions to attempt to do so. No herbal or pharmaceutical company would consider spending that kind of money on an unpatentable medicine. After all, to recoup the outlay it would have to charge more for its product than its rivals – not the best conditions for commercial success. Remember too that there are high profit margins on patentable drugs – not so on unpatentable herbs.

Warnings

Once we accept that the use of herbs is a sound approach to medical treatment, we need to know which ones are recommended for the prevention, or cure, of cancer. Before that, however, a warning is in order. Herbs cannot be presumed to be safe – some, indeed, are poisonous. Pregnant women in particular should not take a herb without consulting a professional. *Anyone* taking a herb should preferably consult a practitioner, but at least read up on it first.

Many herbal preparations can be effective in keeping a cancer in remission – but almost all herbalists say that although the herbs may stop a tumour growing or even shrink it so that it is clinically invisible, they cannot kill the tumour. Once the herbs are no longer being taken, the cancer returns. Diet, they say, is the only way to correct whatever the underlying cause was. On the plus side, on the other hand, because of their biochemical complexity, cancers will not become resistant to herbs as they do to purified chemicals.

189

Astragalus

Astragalus is a Chinese herb used mainly for patients with heart disease or high blood pressure. It has recently been shown to have a very strong normalising effect on people with damaged immune systems. It is therefore not only recommended as a cancer prevention/cure, but also as a herbal support for people undergoing chemotherapy and radiation.

Dose: 1–3 400 mg capsules per day.

Chaparral

Chaparral is a desert plant covering large areas of southern California and Arizona. It has small, brittle leaves, which have been used by the local Indian people to make a health tonic tea. It has a pungent smell and very bitter taste. One dramatic case of a cancer cure using chaparral alone occurred in 1967 to 1968. The patient was an eighty-seven-year-old man by the name of Ernest Farr, who had had four operations on a malignant melanoma and been told there was no point in further surgery. He drank chaparral tea over a period of four months. The cancer shrank almost entirely away and was still very small nine months later. Clearly, something in the chaparral had worked. (At the age of ninety-six, Farr died of the same melanoma. It appears that his doctor had refused to allow him to continue taking chaparral tea.)

Scientists investigated, and found the chemical substance NDGA. This was already a well-known chemical, as it was used to preserve butter in the tropics. It is a very powerful antioxidant. It is not known whether it works for all cancers – one test found little activity against breast cancer, while another found it to be effective against gastro-intestinal cancer.

However, there is a caution. One woman taking chaparral in large quantities suffered severe liver damage. A study has also shown that chaparral taken in very small doses may be counter-effective and result in stimulating the tumour. The same result has, interestingly, also been shown in one Italian study for vitamin C. A little may be a bad thing.

Chaparral can be used as a douche for cervical dysplasia (a teaspoon in 1.1 litres/2 pints of warm water). This approach may work for many of the herbal substances mentioned in this book, for those with cervical cancer.

Dose: Ernest Farr took 7–8 grams of fresh chaparral leaves and steeped them in 1.1 litres (2 pints) hot water. He drank two to three cups a day. As with other herbal cancer cures, chaparral needs to be continued after the tumour appears to have disappeared. Long-term chaparral users need to take iron supplements.

Chinese herbs

The Chinese view tumours as the 'uppermost branch' of the disease, not its root. They consider cancer to be caused by a wide range of external or internal excesses, i.e. an excessive dose of a cancer-causing chemical, or an excessive dose of bad emotions. All forms of excess result in the qi, the body's living energy, becoming blocked in some way.

Some Chinese doctors prefer to treat cancer with herbs alone, while others mix Chinese herbs with chemotherapy and radiation. Fu-zhen therapy, an immune-enhancing herbal regimen, has had very good results when compared with chemotherapy and radiation. In one study of seventy-six patients with stage 2 liver cancer, forty-six were treated with fu-zhen herbs in combination with chemotherapy and radiation. Twenty-nine survived for one year, and ten for three years. Only six of the thirty given chemotherapy and radiation survived one year. In fact, success came from using the herbs alone.

The most commonly used fu-zhen herbs are astragalus, ligustrum, ginseng, codonopsis, atractylodes, ganoderma, actinidia and rabdosia. Actinidia is a root that contains the polysaccharide ACPS-R. In one study, when it was injected into mice, ninety per cent of tumours stopped growing. Another study showed a fifty per cent success rate with liver cancers.

Doctors at the Beijing Institute for Cancer Research have found that a herbal tonic usually prescribed for kidney ailments, known variously as Golden Book Tea or Six Flavour Tea, had a highly significant effect when combined with chemotherapy against small cell lung cancer. It appears that all traditional kidney tonics may have these beneficial effects.

Tang kuei (*Angelica sinensis*) is a highly reputed blood tonic, which has had successful results in treating cancer either alone or in combination with other herbs. Women have used it as a douche against cervical cancer.

Another herb is juzentaihoto, sometimes known as JT-48, or JTT. It is a blood-strengthening herb, which is reportedly very effective in helping chemotherapy patients recover. There are certainly other Chinese herbs that will also be beneficial.

It should be noted that Chinese herbalists have an attitude to the value of a herb that is totally opposed to the way Western doctors view drugs. For a Western doctor, the best kind of drug is one that has a specific effect against a specific ailment. The more generalised a drug's effects, the less it is valued. Any drug that claims to be a cure-all will be automatically disregarded as valueless. For Chinese herbalists, the reverse is true. For them, the most inferior herb is the one that acts against a single specific problem. The most valued is the one that has a broad spectrum of effects. Since herbalists seek first and foremost to promote the total health of an individual, this makes sense.

Most Chinese herb books do not, in fact, list cancer as a disease that herbs can fight. Instead, they note the herbs that are effective in strengthening the immune system. More specific agents may be listed as anti-viral agents.

Studies have shown a very strong supportive effect of Chinese herbs and herbal tonics for patients undergoing surgery, radiation and chemotherapy. Patients taking Chinese herbs live longer and suffer less severe side-effects. Most anti-cancer herbal formulae contain herbs that:

> supplement qi energy
> clear the heat
> regulate the blood
> supplement the blood
> supplement yin
> supplement yang. (Boik, 1995)

Some critics of Chinese-grown herbs point out that China's herbal doctors depend on large quantities of the basic herbs. These cannot be obtained from the wild in the necessary quantities, so have to be grown commercially. The mineral

192

content of most of China's farmlands is heavily depleted, and pesticide use is standard. The result is that herbs are of low potency. Chinese herbs that are grown in Canada, the US or Australia should therefore be obtained.

Mainstream medicine is now going back to its roots with a new series of drugs deriving from herbs and tree barks. Taxol is one (made from the Pacific yew tree). A new one is Campto, derived from a Chinese tree, the xi-shu, or 'tree of happiness'. This latter is having some success with colon cancer. Anyone seeking further information should contact the Royal Marsden Hospital, London.

The Clark cure

The Clark cure, put forward by Dr Hulda Clark, is a new and surprising addition to the herbal armoury – and very radical. Indeed, if she is right, the entire cancer research industry can switch off its lights and go home. Clark's view is that cancer is caused by a parasite – the human intestinal fluke. This causes no major problems in the gut where it normally resides, but by some means as yet unknown – but associated with the presence of propyl alcohol – it can move to other organs, where it starts creating problems. The problem it creates if it gets to the liver is cancer. Her test for cancer is to test for the presence of the chemical marker ortho-phospho-tyrosine.

Just as the cause is simple, so is the cure that Clark proposes: black walnut tincture, wormwood and cloves. The first two kill adult and developmental stages of over one hundred parasites; the cloves kill the eggs.

Dr Hulda Clark is a Canadian physiologist, who published details of her cure with one hundred case studies in her book *The Cure for All Cancers*. She believes that many, if not most, ailments, from asthma and AIDS to heart disease and schizophrenia, are the result of parasitical infection and the formula she gives above is one that she believes will rid the body of many of these. She accepts that other formulas will also work.

In Clark's view, the parasite is only half the problem – the other half is the propyl alcohol. Most people can process this effectively, and so it causes them no problems. But people developing cancer have an impaired ability to do this. For this, she blames the presence in the liver of aflatoxin B. This is a known carcinogenic substance, found in mouldy food.

One way to deal with the problem, she argues, is to eliminate propyl alcohol from the system. Unfortunately, it is a common antiseptic used in the food and cosmetics industries. Check the items in your bathroom, and you will find most contain one of the following ingredients: propanol, isopropyl alcohol, isopropanol, and so on. Even if not listed, Clark claims that propyl alcohol is commonly used for cleaning industrial equipment and so may be present in minute quantities in a wide range of modern retail goods. For those people with an impaired ability to break it down, even these quantities are sufficient to cause cancer. She particularly notes hair and cosmetic products, sugar, carbonated soft drinks and even bottled water, fruit drinks and vitamin supplements. She makes an exception for vitamin C, as this helps the liver to break down propyl alcohol by directly attacking the aflatoxin.

Dose:

1. Black walnut tincture: This should be taken in a glass of water four times a day. Start the first day with one drop each time, and increase the dose by one drop a day until on the twentieth day you are taking twenty drops in water four times a day. Then reduce to twenty drops once a day for three months; then reduce to thirty drops once a day, two days a week. It should be taken on an empty stomach, i.e. half an hour before a meal.

2. Wormwood: This herb is made from the leaves of the Artemesia shrub. It is also available from herbalists as part of a combination of herbs. It should be taken once a day before the evening meal, increasing daily from one capsule to fourteen. Then maintain this level twice a week for life.

3. Cloves: Obtain whole cloves and grind them up – do not use cloves that have already been ground. Fill capsules (preferably, size 00) with the ground cloves and take three times a day before meals, building up from one capsule a time to three capsules a time. Continue until the tenth day, and then reduce to three capsules once a day for three months. Then take just twice a week for life.

Clark's four-point plan for regaining health is simple, but extreme: remove every unnatural chemical substance from your mouth, from your diet, from your body and from your home. This part of her recommendations may be unrealisable. But since the herbal part of her cure is cheap and not harmful, we can happily do this no matter what else we wish to do.

Co-enzyme Q10 (CoQ10)

The quinone family of chemical compounds is a very important one for cancer. One of the major chemotherapeutic drugs, adriamycin, is a quinone. Adriamycin is an oxidative quinone whose effects are very different from others like CoQ10, which are antioxidative. It is therefore dangerous for people with weak hearts. CoQ10 protects against this effect. It is recommended that anyone undergoing chemotherapy with adriamycin should take large amounts of CoQ10.

Co-enzyme Q10 is a quinone found almost everywhere in nature – which is why it is called the ubiquitous quinone, ubiquinone for short. But it is present in extremely small quantities – too small to be medically useful. While many quinones have an improved immuno-strengthening effect at very small doses, ubiquinone is not one of these. CoQ10 has an increased effect with larger doses. It is known that people with cancer have reduced levels of CoQ10, suggesting that it is used up in fighting the tumour.

Dose: A Danish study, published in 1994, found that women with terminal breast cancer did very well when taking 390 mg a day. This amount seemed to be sufficient to prevent further tumour growth, and even to cause tumour shrinkage. A group of thirty-two women with advanced stage breast cancer were given, in addition to the normal treatments of surgery, radiation and chemotherapy, a programme of supplements, including 390 mg of CoQ10.

Unfortunately, CoQ10 is not readily absorbed into the body on its own, so it needs to be taken in conjunction with other substances. CoQ10 should be mixed with borage or flax oil, with the contents of one high dose vitamin E capsule and 300 mg of L-cysteine (an amino acid). This should be taken as part of a programme known as the Stockholm Protocol, which was used by researcher Knut Lockwood. Lockwood found it effective in stabilising and eliminating tumours, even in cases where breast cancer had metastasised to the liver – an extraordinary finding. The full daily Stockholm Protocol is as follows:

- GLA (borage or evening primrose oil)   1.2 grams
- Omega 3 fatty acids (flax oil)   3.5 grams
- Beta-carotene capsules   32,000 iu
- Vitamin C   3 grams
- Vitamin E   2,500 iu
- Selenium   400 mcg
- Co-enzyme Q10   390 mcg

The following is also recommended for liver support; for every 50 lb or 22.5 kg of body weight, three times a day:

- 300 mg alpha lipoic acid
- 300 mg curcumin
- 300 mg milk thistle extract

The vitamin C used by Lockwood was a combination of calcium, magnesium and potassium ascorbates. It is the experience of others that calcium ascorbate is either useless or dangerous. The ideal mix should include sodium, zinc, magnesium and potassium ascorbates.[19]

Essiac

Essiac is another Canadian herbal treatment for cancer, and one that similarly has caused controversy. The official story of Essiac starts in 1922, when a young nurse by the name of Rene Caisse was given the names of a number of herbs by an old woman who had cured herself of breast cancer by drinking a herbal tea. This old woman had got the remedy from a native Ojibwa Indian. Some time later, Caisse's aunt was diagnosed with terminal stomach cancer and given six months to live. With the doctor's consent, Caisse gave the herbs to her aunt – who went on to live another twenty-one years. She was then given more cases, and these also healed. Caisse not only gave the Essiac combination (named by

196

reversing her own name) in the form of tea, but also – in a modified form – by injection in the site of the cancer, which she found to be quicker and more effective

Doctors were so impressed that they petitioned the Canadian government in 1926 to give Rene Caisse facilities for research. The result? They tried to arrest her for treating cancer without a medical licence. Fortunately, Caisse had the support of nine very eminent doctors, so the government desisted. Gradually, however, official disapproval tightened the noose and doctors, fearing for their own careers, started to distance themselves from her. In 1938, a Commission of Enquiry conducted an investigation. Unlike Mary Johnson, Rene Caisse did not receive a generous appraisal. It concluded that of all the patients who came to testify on her behalf, none had ever had cancer – despite their X-rays and medical documentation.

Rene Caisse continued to give patients her herbal treatment – without making any charge. In one case, she records that her treatment for cancer had the interesting side-effect of also curing the patient's diabetes. If, as Dr Clark believes, diabetes is also caused by a parasitical fluke, then Essiac may work by eliminating the parasites.

There are currently a number of variations on the market – Essiac, Tea of Life, Flor-Essence and possibly others – but they all share the same official ingredients: burdock root, Turkish rhubarb, slippery elm and sheep sorrel. Additional ingredients found in commercial Essiac teas are: red clover blossom, kelp, blessed thistle herb and watercress herb. The tea can be drunk both as a treatment for cancer or as a preventative health tonic.

Rene Caisse died in 1978, at the age of ninety-one. In 1983, Bruce Hendrick, Chief of the Division of Neurosurgery at the Hospital for Sick Children in Toronto, wrote to the Canadian Minister for Health and Welfare asking her to authorise clinical trials on the effectiveness of Essiac tea. In his letter he said: 'I am most impressed with the effectiveness of the treatment and its lack of side-effects.' Further support for its effectiveness comes from Dr Charles Brusch, once personal physician to former US President John F. Kennedy, who also claims to have been cured of his cancer using Essiac.

The Canadian Cancer Society nevertheless considers Essiac to be a questionable, or at least unproven, method of cancer treatment. Canadian health laws prohibit it from being marketed as an anti-cancer treatment; however, it is available on prescription, although the prescribing doctor must first get authorisation from the Deputy Director of the Health Protection branch.

CAUTIONS
Essiac may cause some nausea or diarrhoea. The Canadian authorities also warn that it is not established that the commercial brands named above are in fact made with the true Essiac recipe. Nevertheless, the manufacturers of Flor-Essence and Tea of Life are able to produce testimonial letters from people who claim to have been cured by the herbal tea. One of the main constituents – burdock root – has demonstrated anti-tumour activity on its own but, as with all herbal formulas, it is the synergistic effects that are important and which remain largely unexplored.[20]

European herbs
The following herbs are proposed by Maria Treben, an Austrian herbalist, and Dr Vogel, an internationally renowned Swiss herbalist, as being good for cancer. None of these herbs have negative side-effects, and can be taken in large quantities.

Horsetail (*Equisetum arvense*): This is one of the most ancient of cancer cures. The horsetail can be used in the form of a tea or a poultice. Horsetail is rich in silica.

Calendula (*Marigold*): A fresh juice of the whole plant – leaves, stem and flower – should be drunk regularly.

Yarrow (*Milfoil, Achillea millefolium*): This is especially recommended for women.

Stinging nettle: The whole plant is used. It has a great reputation for blood cleansing. Pick them in May, and store for the winter.

Butterbur (*Petasites officinalis, hybridus*): This is highly recommended both as a cancer treatment and as a pain reliever. It is the basis of Vogel's herbal product, Petaforce.

Maria Treben recommends for a general cancer treatment a tea made as follows:

300 g (11 oz) calendula
100 g (3½ oz) yarrow
100 g (3½ oz) stinging nettle
2 litres (3½ pints) water

Place the fresh herbs in a non-metallic teapot or other container. Bring the water to the boil and pour over the herbs. Steep for half a minute or so – the tea should be light yellow or green in colour. (Dried herbs are steeped for one to two minutes.)

For leukaemia, she recommends a tea consisting of:

15 g (½ oz) St John's Wort and dandelion roots
20 g (¾ oz) speedwell and wormwood
25 g (1 oz) bedstraw, yarrow and goat's beard
30 g (1¼ oz) elder shoots, calendula, greater celandine and stinging nettle

Mix all the ingredients together. Place 1 heaped teaspoon in a cup, and pour boiling water over it. Leave for a half to two minutes (longer with dried herbs, shorter time with fresh). Make 1–2 litres (1¾–3½ pints) for a day. Keep in a thermos and sip. (One cup is 250 ml or a quarter litre.)

Hoxsey's herbs

In 1840, one John Hoxsey had a horse with a cancerous growth. Thinking there was nothing he could do, he turned the horse loose on a pasture. Amazingly, the cancerous growth soon began to shrink, and eventually it fell off. Hoxsey observed the horse and saw that it liked to go to a certain part of the pasture and graze on the plants there. If we accept that all animals have an instinct for healing plants, then there is nothing strange about this story. Hoxsey collected the plants from that part of his field, and experimented with them in various combinations. Eventually, he made a formula that was handed down from father to son until it reached Harry Hoxsey in 1919.

Harry Hoxsey began opening cancer clinics around the USA. He had seventeen when the cancer establishment started to crack down. Eventually, after being arrested 125 times in sixteen months, for practising medicine without a licence, Hoxsey was forced to close down. The cases were,

199

however, all thrown out of court. In 1963, his chief nurse opened the Bio-medical Centre in Tijuana, Mexico, where Hoxsey's herbal treatment is still available.

Hoxsey's Herbs contains the following: red clover (*Trifolium pratense*), burdock root (*Arctium lappa*), licorice (*Glycyrrhiza glabra*), Oregon grape root (*Mahonia repens*), Cascara sagrada (*Rhamnus purshiana*), buckthorn (*Rhamnus frangula*), poke root (*Phtolacca decandra*), prickly ash (*Xanthoxylum americanum*), wild indigo (*Baptisia tinctoria*) with potassium iodide. Chaparral (*Larrea tridentata*) is apparently a late addition to the formula.

Patricia Spain, who did a study of the herbs for the US Congress Office of Technology as part of its assessment of alternative cancer therapies, wrote in her report: 'More recent literature leaves no doubt that Hoxsey's formula does indeed contain many plant substances of marked therapeutic activity.'

Pau d'arco and cat's claw
In 1967, the Brazilian newspaper *O'Cruzeiro* reported the story of a cancer-stricken girl from Rio de Janeiro who continually prayed for a cure. In a dream or vision, she saw a monk who told her that she would recover if she made a tea brewed with the bark of the pau d'arco tree. The monk returned in a second vision and told her which specific pau d'arco trees she was to use. Whether these visions were true – perhaps a response to a subconscious recognition of the medicinal powers of this tree – or whether they were simply a necessary guise in which to cloak a desire persuasively, the girl was given the tea she required – and she recovered. She was not alone. Many others have claimed their cancers have gone into long-term remission after drinking pau d'arco tea.

Anecdotal evidence and folk practice throughout South America appears to justify the claims made for this tree bark. Besides cancer, it is supposedly effective against diabetes, ulcers and rheumatism, to name a few. The bark of the tree contains many chemicals that are known to have anti-tumour effects: tannins, quinones and triterpines and others. There are many different varieties of the pau d'arco tree – and each variety seems to have its own range of medicinal characteristics. Its anti-cancer effects have been demonstrated in a number of animal studies.

200

Pau d'arco – also known as lapacho and taheebo – is available as a bark, in powdered form and as an alcoholic extract. Unfortunately, most studies on the alcoholic extracts commercially available in Europe and North America consider them to be medically useless, as they do not appear to contain the active ingredient, lapachol. Others argue that looking for a single active ingredient is wrong; pau d'arco contains at least twelve quinones, of which lapachol is only one. Pau d'arco pills are also not considered useful. The tea barks themselves vary in quality, some having no measurable lapachol. However, lapachol is an effective immunostimulator in extremely low quantities, so the barks may be effective even though the presence of lapachol is not evident.

A tea is made by boiling six tablespoons bark in four cups boiling water. Boil the water until it reduces to three cups. This takes about five minutes. The tea is then cooled and filtered. Three to eight cups a day should be taken, each cup sipped slowly but steadily. The remainder should be kept refrigerated. Toxicity is low. The symptom to expect from over-consumption is a slight skin rash.

Another South American herb believed to have powerful anti-cancer properties is *Uncaria tomentosa*, known as cat's claw. Again, there appears to be little danger of toxicity. High doses are recommended for cancer patients.

Reishi mushrooms

The Japanese call it 'reishi', the Chinese 'ling zhi'. It was highly revered by Taoists in search of the elixir of immortality. Of course, any herb associated with long life is likely to have shown clear evidence of general medicinal value. There are a number of varieties, the most potent of which is considered by the Chinese to be the red fungus – but this may simply be because the colour red has a positive symbolism in Chinese culture. Reishi mushrooms are very high in polysaccharides, which may be responsible for their effect of stimulating the immune system. The Chinese view reishi as a tonic that boosts the vital life energy, or qi.

Studies have shown that reishi mushroom extract can kill stapphylococci and streptococci bacteria. This makes it a very useful treatment for pneumonia and hospital-acquired infections. Interestingly, low doses of the mushroom appear to be more effective than large ones. The optimal dose appears to be 4 grams a day. One Japanese cancer surgeon, Dr Fukumi Morishige, stumbled on this by chance when a woman who was dying of cancer suddenly appeared to be cured. Morishige discovered that her husband had been giving her fresh reishi mushroom tea every day. Morishige now prescribes a daily intake of 4 grams of reishi tea, with 10 grams of a special form of vitamin C known as nucleic acid ascorbate.

Morishige discovered that large doses of vitamin C prevented the diarrhoea caused by taking in too much reishi. He therefore reasoned that the vitamin C was having the effect of increasing its absorbability. In this way, he was able to increase the reishi dose to 9 grams a day. Now, doses of 9–15 grams ($1/4$-$1/2$ oz) a day are standard in the US. Reishi can also be taken effectively by intravenous injection. Morishige has treated and cured a number of cancer patients using nothing else but this combination of vitamin C and reishi mushrooms.

Studies undertaken by the National Cancer Research Centre show that mice injected with reishi extract showed tumour regression between fifty and one hundred per cent, depending on the dose.

People who take reishi mushrooms show a marked increase in blood oxygenation levels, and for this reason reishi is also used as an antidote to altitude sickness. The importance in cancer treatment of having high tissue oxygen levels has already been mentioned, and this may be one of the ways in which reishi has an anti-cancer effect. Apart from its claimed anti-cancer effects, it is recommended in Japan for patients undergoing radiation and chemotherapy, as a way of reducing side-effects.

Some healers use reishi in combination with shiitake mushrooms and astragalus.

It can have a few unpleasant side-effects – dizziness, light-headedness and itchiness. These can be dealt with by lowering the dose and then slowly increasing it. There have been no signs of toxicity in many studies, even up to levels equivalent to a human taking 350 grams (12 oz) a day.

Reishi is very bitter and is not eaten as a food. It is cut into pieces and brewed in hot water: 5 grams ($1/5$ oz) per 1 litre ($1 3/4$ pints). The water is simmered until it is reduced to a third of a litre (about 10 fl oz). It is then drunk. The vitamin C has to be taken separately as it is destroyed by heat. Reishi is also available in capsule form. At present it is quite expensive, and as a result a great deal of fake ling zhi has made its way on to the market.

Triterpines

This is a family of essential oils found in many plants, which seem to be the most potent ingredient in many herbs and plant extracts associated with longevity. And, of course, long life can be seen simply as a life not shortened by cancer. The following are known to contain significant quantities of triterpines: Siberian ginseng, licorice root, gingko leaves, gotu kola (a creeping herb, common in India), soybeans and chaga (a Russian herb used as an anti-cancer agent). These herbs have shown significant anti-tumour activity in studies in the US and Finland. Olives contain oleanolic acid, a triterpine, which is being examined with great interest by the Japanese as a chemopreventive of cancer.

Ayurvedic medicine

This 6,000-year-old Indian therapy uses a wide range of herbal and other treatments, but because of its complexity, it cannot usefully be summarised here. As with Chinese herbalists, it is recognised that a single cancer may arise from different causes, and therefore needs to be treated accordingly. As an indication of what is possible with Ayurveda, we can consider the case study presented in 1989 to the Indian Association of Cancer Chemotherapists. Dr Joshi, an allopathic doctor who also uses Ayurvedic methods, reported on 422 terminal cancer patients he had treated since 1973. Of these, seventeen per cent obtained complete relief of their symptoms and 'prolongation of life'. Partial relief of symptoms occurred in 292 cases (sixty-nine per cent) and there was no response in twenty-one per cent. For an introduction to Ayurveda, see Deepak Chopra, *Perfect Health*.

Bloodroot

Bloodroot is a herb which according to some observers has demonstrated very powerful anti-cancer properties. Bloodroot, *Sanguinaria canadensis*, is native to the woods of north-central United States and Canada. Its taproot exudes a blood-coloured juice, from which its name derives. It was one of the most popular herbal remedies among Plains Indians, who used it internally for sore throats and respiratory ailments and externally for growths on the surface of the body. It is this last property that makes it interesting for cancer patients – especially for those with melanoma or other surface tumours. Quite simply, it dissolves any form of malignant growth while leaving healthy tissue alone.

Dr Andrew Weil used some bloodroot on his dog, which was suffering from a large surface tumour. For three days, he smeared a thin layer of paste on the tumour. He stopped on the fourth day, because he was alarmed to see blood. It seemed that the tumour was separating itself from the flesh around it. He disinfected the wound and kept an eye on developments. Two days later the entire tumour fell off and the raw flesh around it quickly healed up.

Here, then, is a herb that directly attacks cancers. Its effects are enhanced by mixing it with zinc chloride. It forms a scab over the cancer and expels it from the body. No secondary infections follow. It is possible that the bloodroot will seek out tumours and eliminate them even when they are not on the surface.

Unfortunately, the ointment used by Dr Weil is extremely difficult to get hold of because of the excessive vigilance of the Food and Drug Administration (FDA) in the US. The supplier is now believed to be living in Nassau, in the Bahamas. We are not free to have access to bloodroot. The very few people 'in the know' will quietly seek out this treatment for themselves, but the vast majority of cancer patients will be deprived of this source of hope. Does this make sense as public policy? Clearly not, yet it will remain policy until there is effective pressure for change.

A mixture of herbs with bloodroot as the main ingredient is available in the USA, but finding the right source is not easy. One solution is to approach your local herbalist, who may be able to make up an ointment containing the following ingredients: water, zinc chloride, bloodroot paste, glycerin, galanga, capsicum, burdock, larrea and urea. See Resources for another possible source.[21]

The manufacturer of the ointment as used by Dr Weil also markets an oral version, called Cansema Tonic. This contains the following listed ingredients: distilled water, alcohol, chaparral, red clover, taheebo bark, inkberry, galangal root, bloodroot, arrowroot, zinc chloride, unrefined, unprocessed honey and glycerine. One teaspoon may be taken in a cup of water – with meals, as it may cause nausea.

CAUTION
Bloodroot ointment is extremely caustic. It must not be ingested, it must be kept away from children and it should not be applied close to any mucous membranes – mouth, eyes, rectum or genitalia. The ointment should be applied in very small doses, as large doses can cause severe burning, nausea and sleeplessness.

Saw palmetto
This is the herb for anyone with prostate problems. It is also supposed to have aphrodisiac properties, which is good, as regular sexual activity is supposed to be beneficial for men with prostate disease. When purchasing this herb, ensure that the strength is eighty-five to ninety-five per cent fatty acids and sterols. Take 160 mg twice daily.

In addition, those with prostate cancer should take zinc (50–60 mg a day), because their prostate fluids are low in this mineral. In one study, fourteen out of nineteen patients treated with zinc showed tumour shrinkage. Magnesium has also been shown to be beneficial for the prostate.

Other herbs
The following herbs have been shown to have a strong general anti-cancer effect, and also to be protective against the adverse effects of radiation: cumin, poppy seeds, ambrosia and fo-ti. Of benefit to the liver are milk thistle, artichoke, dandelion, turmeric and rosemary.

Chlorophyll has shown a marked ability to prevent or slow the development of cancerous mutations according to studies at MD Anderson Hospital in Houston, Texas. Since it is abundant in green vegetables (the darker the better), there is no problem of access. Chlorophyll is chemically almost identical to haemoglobin, and this seems to support the value of using Chinese herbal blood-strengthening tonics for cancer patients.

For information on sources for herbs, see Resources.[22]

Cancer and the mind

Psychotherapy and cancer-prone personalities

One of the first investigators into the field of psychology and cancer was Dr Lawrence LeShan, an experimental psychologist and therapist. Starting in the 1950s in America, he undertook research into whether there were psychological predisposing characteristics which might explain why some people got cancer – and whether this could be used to help people to recover. This research spanned three decades, and his conclusions were 'yes' to both questions.

LeShan quotes the case of 'John', who had a massive, inoperable brain tumour. After working with LeShan using a special form of psychotherapy – which LeShan characterises as 'crisis therapy' – John recovered without medication, even though his doctors had told him he had only months to live. John's psychological state before he met LeShan was one of hopelessness. After going through psychotherapy, he developed a much more positive frame of mind. His attitude to life turned around, and his terminal cancer disappeared.

In his book, *You Can Fight for Your Life*, LeShan described the process by which John and a number of other patients underwent complete remission. He also argued that even those he worked with who died from their cancers nevertheless had the quality of their lives dramatically transformed for the better through his therapy.

LeShan's work began when he and a co-worker discovered that there seemed to be startling similarities in the personality configurations and life histories of people who subsequently died of cancer – a personality configuration very similar to that of people with a predisposition to suicide. LeShan believed that if there were such a configuration, it should be tracked down.

In the first stage of his research, LeShan interviewed 250

patients – spending between two and eight hours with each one. Another 200 cancer patients were interviewed for specific concerns. Close relatives of over fifty patients were interviewed for between one and three hours, and another forty close relatives were seen for between twenty and fifty hours. This was over a period of fourteen years. In addition, he undertook intensive psychotherapy with seventy-one patients.

As a result of his study, LeShan came to the conclusions that:

1. 'There is a general type of personality configuration among the majority of cancer patients.'
2. 'People whose personality or life history conforms to this pattern of susceptibility can take steps to protect themselves against the possibility of cancer.'

What LeShan discovered was that for a significant majority of cancer cases there had been, prior to the onset of cancer, a loss of a crucial relationship. This loss may have been a physical or, more frequently, an emotional loss – for instance, the failure of a marriage, or a marriage from which the heart had gone, or an attachment to a way of life or activity that promised happiness but which was then denied to the person for some reason. From this perception, he predicted that age-corrected cancer rates for women would be highest for widows, next highest for divorced women, then for married women without children, followed by married women with children and lowest for single women. Epidemiological statistics from various sources appear to support this conclusion.

He found that for a large majority of cancer patients there is a clear inability to express hostility, anger or resentment. He went on to discover that cancers developed in people who were in despair because they frustrated their own creative potential. They denied themselves. They felt that they had to be other than themselves to be accepted, and conversely that they would be rejected by others if they were themselves.

LeShan's patient, John, had become a lawyer and joined his father's firm as a result of strong parental suggestion; he had married a woman who enjoyed being the wife of a lawyer and had been chosen by his parents. However, he was deeply dissatisfied. As a child, John had shown a great deal of interest in music and had dreamed of being a pianist. As a result of his therapy, John came to accept that it was possible for him to be a pianist if he really wanted to, and that he had a right to fight for what he wanted. He quit his job, divorced his wife, took up the piano seriously and eventually became a pianist with a symphony orchestra. His terminal brain cancer disappeared.

While many people feel despair, LeShan discovered that the despair of the cancer patient has unique features: 'The patient in despair is absolutely alone. At the deepest emotional level he cannot relate, since he does not believe himself worthy of love. He does not despair over "something", as would the usual depressed patient – rather, he despairs over "nothing".'

Trapped in this alone-ness, the cancer patient is in an emotional place where it is impossible to be reached by love, where any kind of fulfilling or satisfying relationship becomes impossible. The cancer patient is even divorced from such negative emotions as anger, resentment and jealousy. As one of his patients said to LeShan: 'You don't understand, doctor. It's not that I've been or done anything. It's that I've done nothing and been nothing.'

'The cancer patient's own desires and wishes had been so completely repressed, that when at the start of the therapy I asked the question "What do you really want out of life?" the response would be a blank and astonished stare. That question had never been seen as valid.'

This despair was evident in sixty-eight out of the seventy-one patients he worked with. LeShan believed strongly that patients feeling this level of despair could be helped, and his case studies showed that he succeeded. He does not give statistics in his book regarding the number of remissions that resulted among the patients; but, in addition to John, he mentions four other patients who recovered, without medication, from terminal cancer.

Remission of cancer among terminal cases is considered extremely rare. One in 100,000 has been one estimate. Yet LeShan is implicitly claiming to have achieved an inconceivably higher success rate. One of the reasons LeShan gives no statistics is because he does not want remission of cancer to be the only yardstick of value. Indeed, LeShan believes that many of those he worked with rediscovered themselves and led lives that were worth living – after decades of failing to do that. As one of his patients said: 'Death is nothing. It is inevitable. Everyone has to die. What matters is how you live and die.'

And it wasn't just the patient who was affected by the course of the patient's psychotherapy. The daughter of one patient wrote to LeShan after her mother had died: 'I know that every day she grew in courage and understanding, and was learning to fight the fears that surrounded her. My father and I are changed, and I think it influenced her friends who visited her. Mother's last months were filled with hope and thoughts of the future.' This is why LeShan is not concerned to boast about success rates on a simple cure/death ratio. Success can be measured qualitatively. It was the objective of his therapy to 'reawaken the inner life of the individual, and to liberate those forces which can enable the person to experience as completely as possible both himself and the meaning of his life and death'.

The crisis therapy that LeShan developed is very different from orthodox psychotherapy. Firstly, it dispenses with the view that unconscious forces rigidly control a helpless ego. He believes that the individual can be freed from constrictions to create his or her own world, and to express his or her own true feelings. He also believes that this demands absolute honesty and openness from the therapist – the therapist does not allow him/herself to have an unexpressed commentary flowing in parallel to the therapy session. Everything must be made explicit. Time is short, and the past needs to be confronted if the therapy is to succeed. This honesty must permeate the relationship, and it precludes kindness – which LeShan sees as a protective device for the therapist, and implying a superior position. The crisis therapist must be in full personal contact with the patient, otherwise he is simply conspiring to avoid the key issues that underlie the cancer. 'Death, the figure in the background, asks the questions, and the therapist must join in the search for answers that are meaningful to the patient.'

The crisis therapist also talks to the family, to prepare them for change – because they are a constraining factor, whether or not they intend to be. This requires a great deal of support and cooperation from the family.

And what is the goal of this therapy? To make patients confront their true selves, to become aware of their real desires, and to make them feel important to themselves. In the mirror of death, some patients feel free to explore this question. Anyone seeking psychotherapy because of cancer should discuss LeShan's ideas with the therapist at the first meeting. This will establish the foundations of the relationship.

Self-help

LeShan favours the idea of psychological self-help, and suggests two useful techniques – one to confront the past, the other the future.

To confront the past, LeShan suggests the following technique. In the darkness of the imagination, we can enter a time machine and return as adults to the critical times in our pasts, the times that can still cause us pain, the times when the seeds of the present – perhaps the self's self-denial – were sown, and face the child that was ourselves then. And when we are there, adult and child, face to face, we should think what we would like to say to that child. This kind of self-confronting journey has a very powerful potential to heal psychic wounds.

For those who feel helpless in the face of the future, LeShan suggests a second technique: the person should focus on an apparently impossible ambition, and then ask himself: 'What is the first thing that has to be done, the very first thing, to achieve this goal?' Every journey starts with a single step. If that first step is taken, there is a good chance the journey will be completed. Without that step, there is no journey.

People who are self-determining, LeShan argues, do not get cancer (or are very much less likely to). People who discover and embrace a purpose can cure themselves of cancer, even when medical science has done everything it can do and fails. If they aren't cured, at least every minute of life left to them is enhanced in value.

Mind-body interaction

One of the imponderable facts about cancer is that some are aggressive, developing very quickly, while others are slow

210

and steady in their development. LeShan believes the aggressiveness is a direct reflection of the speed at which the cancer occurs after the loss of life's meaning, as embodied in a central relationship. That is to say, the cause of an aggressive cancer is to be found shortly before the cancer develops, while the cause of a slow-growing cancer is to be found further in the past. The psychologist, Dr Bruno Klopfer, claimed to be able to predict with eighty per cent accuracy which patients had slow-growing cancers, and which fast growing, on the basis of personality tests alone. Those with the more acutely felt despair had the more aggressive cancers.

LeShan and Klopfer seem to be saying that cancer is an accurate measure of despair. This can only be true if the mind and body are inextricably entwined. This matter is a very contentious one. Traditional Western philosophy and science are based on the assumption that mind and body are separate. The mind is even seen as distinct from the brain, the physical organ associated with it. If they are distinct and separate, how can one affect the other? If a doctor says: 'It's psychosomatic – it's all in the mind,' he is saying it isn't real, that it only exists as a thought, not as a fact. Against this view is the one – widely accepted in ancient times, and also today by many other cultures – that mind and body are one, inextricable whole: what affects the body affects the mind, and vice versa.

The idea that emotions can cause cancer is a common one and indeed for most of the last 2,000 years – with the sole exception of the twentieth century – it was the standard view. At the end of the nineteenth century, Sir James Paget, one of the leading medical figures of his time, reflected the orthodox view when he wrote: 'The cases are so frequent in which deep anxiety, deferred hope and disappointment are quickly followed by the growth and increase of cancer that we can hardly doubt that mental depression is a weighty additive to the other influences favouring the development of the cancerous constitution.'

It is only in this century, with its overemphasis on the mechanical features of the body, that the individual's self and his values, beliefs and feelings have been almost totally ignored. Modern medicine deals with the body as if it were a machine. Each bit and piece can be taken out, replaced or

211

tinkered with. People don't die of broken hearts or despair any more; they die of cerebral haemorrhage or cancer of the cervix. The result is that doctors believe it is for them to decide what repair is needed. And if excision of the rectum appears to be necessary for the further functioning of the body-machine, so be it. There is little concern for whether the patient wishes to live with the continuing pain, inconvenience and indignity that such an operation bequeaths.

Yet the great things in life: love, laughter, beauty, courage, as well as the negative things such as fear, worry and danger, belong as much to the mind as to the chemistry of the body. If mind and body are so separate, then why do we cry when we are sad or in pain? Why do we feel a physical thrill at the sight of great beauty? Why do we jump immediately we sense danger? In each of these cases, the physical response does not wait for the conscious message, it is synchronised with the mental message. Mental and physical responses are two sides of a coin that cannot be separated from each other.

We can conclude from this that all thoughts *are* facts. If our mind and body are one, then our body is intelligent and our thoughts are physical. Similarly, if the body is diseased in some way, then we cannot say that we have the disease but rather that the disease is part of us, part of our identity. We are the disease.

This is the belief of Deepak Chopra, a distinguished doctor-writer trained in the West, and who has turned to Ayurvedic medicine. The point of contact between the mind and body are the neuro-peptide transmitters – the body's 'messenger molecules', as Chopra calls them: 'A neuro-peptide springs into existence at the touch of a thought, but where does it spring from? A thought of fear and the neuro-chemical that it turns into are somehow connected to a hidden process, a transformation of non-matter into matter.' Chopra calls the zone where this occurs the '? zone'. This question-mark zone is a place below the visible. It is a world where quantum rules dictate reality – and one of the rules is that things can happen suddenly, absolutely and inexplicably – the so-called quantum leap, where A can become B instantaneously.

Chopra gives an example of such a quantum cure taking place. A patient of his, a woman in her fifties, went to see him complaining of severe abdominal pains and jaundice. He thought at first that she was suffering from gallstones and arranged for surgery, but when she was opened up, it was found that she had a large malignant tumour that had spread to her liver, with scattered pockets of cancer throughout her abdominal cavity. The surgeons considered the cancer to be inoperable and closed the incision without taking further action. Chopra spoke to the woman's daughter first. She pleaded with him not to tell her mother the truth, which Chopra agreed to. He informed the woman that the gallstone operation had been completely successful. He expected her to die within a few months, but eight months later she appeared before him for a routine examination that revealed no signs of cancer. Much later, the woman said to him: 'Doctor, I was so sure I had cancer two years ago that when it turned out to be just gallstones, I told myself I would never be sick another day in my life.'

We can call an event like this a miracle, a spontaneous remission, a placebo cure. But the fact is, whatever words we give it – it happens.

The power of the placebo

A three-year-old boy with a severe case of whooping cough was seen by the doctor. The doctor appeared before the boy in great robes. He sat on the boy's bed and peeled a peach. Then he sugared it and cut it into small pieces. He fed each piece slowly to the boy. As he did so, he told the boy that he was going to be fine, as the peaches would make him well again. He made the boy feel that the return of his health was inevitable. However, on leaving the room he told the father that he did not hold out much hope for the boy. The whooping cough was so serious, it was almost certain to be fatal.

The next day, the boy was still alive, and the doctor came again. As before, he made sure he was wearing his impressive medical robes. As before, he fed the boy with some fruit. After forty days and forty visits, the boy was well again. The doctor was the famous Sir William Osler, and the boy was the brother of Dr Patrick Mallam, who published the story in the *Journal of the American Medical Association* (22 December, 1969). Osler, incidentally, is famous for his comment: 'In today's system of medicine a

213

patient has to recover twice: once from the disease and once from the treatment.'

Just believing that a pill is a powerful pain-reliever can be enough to get rid of the pain in thirty to sixty per cent of the people given a placebo. We can therefore conclude that the level of faith in a therapy helps to determine how successful that therapy is. Curiously, it is not the least educated and those of lower intelligence who are most susceptible to this effect – rather, it is the reverse. Placebos have a higher tendency to work with the more intelligent and educated. And it doesn't appear to be a conscious decision, as placebos don't work because we consciously want them to work. The basis of the placebo's action lies deeper in the mind.

ARE PLACEBOS EFFECTIVE – AND ARE THEY BEING USED?

A number of studies have shown placebos to be thirty to forty per cent effective. That the placebo effect may be even stronger is indicated by some further studies. One showed that valium was more effective than a placebo for the first week of therapy only. After that, they had equal effectiveness. This contradicts the prevalent view that placebo cures are short-lasting. Another study substituted saline solution for morphine with morphine-addicted patients who were being withdrawn from their addiction. No withdrawal symptoms appeared until the saline injections were stopped. The placebo effect is clearly reinforced when the attitude of the doctor is positive.

If we can believe a disease or a pain away, then we can believe it into existence – not consciously perhaps, but at some level of awareness. If the body is intelligent, then it is intelligent in its every part, every organ, every cell. Is this really true – or is it just poetic overstatement? Consider the famous case of a child named Timmy, who suffers from multiple personality disorder. Nearly a dozen personalities contend within his physical frame. One of these personalities is allergic to orange juice, but the allergic reaction stops as soon as another personality takes over.

For this to make sense, we have to accept that the cells of the antibodies that trigger the allergic reaction make a choice as to whether to react. This choice is dependent on the mind's decision about which personality it is at any

214

moment. This means the mind is capable of choosing to be allergic or not allergic. If it can choose to have an allergy, it can also choose to have cancer. If the disease is something we have unconsciously chosen, then the cure too can be chosen.

Given the obvious benefits of placebos, you would think that more would be done with them. Instead, many hospitals present patients with a physical environment that is not conducive to positive thoughts of cure. Often this is because of financial constraints, but the fact is that hospitals and doctors seem to be working against placebos rather than with them. The wise patient will create his or her own placebo-enhancing mental environment.

The reverse process is also true. Many patients, told that their cancer is incurable, promptly fulfil their doctor's expectations by dying. But the example of tuberculosis is instructive. One hundred years ago, this disease had the same fearful prognosis as cancer today; then a cure was found, and death rates dropped sharply – even though most of those who recovered had not yet received the new antibiotic.

The power of expectation is so strong that there are good reasons for not pursuing any form of treatment towards which you have a negative attitude. The Simontons, a husband and wife team, conducted an eighteen-month study with 152 patients into the importance of attitude in determining the outcome of treatment with radiation. The results were clear. Patients with positive attitudes had a better response to the radiation treatment than those with negative attitudes. In fact, of the 152 patients, only two who had shown a negative attitude had a good response to treatment. Patients with a good attitude and a more developed cancer generally did better than patients with a negative attitude but less advanced cancer. This leads to a very important conclusion: cancer patients should only undertake treatments that they are positive about. If you feel that the best place to deal with cancer is in hospital, and that the best weapons are radiation and chemotherapy, then concentrate your thoughts on these. If you feel they will not help, then avoid them.

One of the classic cases of placebo cure was reported by Dr Bruno Klopfer. One of his patients took a drug called krebiozen, and his growths 'melted like snowballs'. A few months later, newspapers reported that the drug was worthless, and the patient's tumours promptly recurred. Suspecting that the patient had a powerful belief system, Klopfer announced that he would give him a more active form of the drug. In fact, he injected his patient with nothing more than distilled water; once again, the tumours disappeared. After a few more months, there were further reports announcing that krebiozen was useless. The patient accepted the truth of these reports, his tumours reappeared, and he quickly died.

A fighting attitude
A study at King's College Hospital, London, looked at the impact of a fighting spirit on the survival of women who had mastectomies for early-stage breast cancer. Ten years later, fifty-five per cent of the group who had the strongest fighting spirit – or whose levels of denial were so strong that they refused to believe they had the disease – had survived, compared with only twenty-two per cent of the group who felt hopeless and helpless, or who stoically accepted their fate.

A hopeful attitude also allowed researchers to predict which women out of sixty-eight who came to a hospital for a cervical biopsy would have cancer. Before the results of the biopsy were known, the women were interviewed and assessed for personality factors. The researchers then predicted who would and who would not have cancer. Of the women who were tested, twenty-eight had cancer. The researchers correctly predicted sixty-eight per cent of the cancer victims and seventy-seven per cent of the cancer-free women simply on the basis of their relative hopefulness, or hopelessness.

In other studies, the degree of hope, faith and trust in a surgeon has been shown to correlate highly with speedier recovery. Curiously, people who avoid thinking about the outcome of an operation recover faster than those who are eternally vigilant. This is further demonstration of a simple truth: that the unconscious is more powerful than the conscious.

Clearly, the mind is capable of unleashing very powerful forces that can lead to both good health and illness. People can will themselves to death and they can will themselves to health. How can we harness these powers? Some methods will already have suggested themselves. Hypnosis, visualisation, and meditation are some of the ways people have recommended. These and other approaches are detailed in An A-Z of alternative options (page 219).

Spiritual consciousness

Some cancer patients go beyond an earth-bound, mind-body nexus. For them, the disease is the key they need to unlock the secret of themselves. They embrace their disease and take responsibility for their response to it. Like a smack over the head from a Zen master, the diagnosis of cancer changes their awareness of – and attitude to – life. One such ex-cancer patient is Petrea King. She believes that her own bout of leukaemia was in some sense psychologically preordained: 'I didn't think "Ah yes, a good dose of leukaemia with a short prognosis is just what I need right now." Yet I firmly believe, at some more subtle level, that the particular disease and prognosis were precisely tailor-made for me.'

The eighteen months preceding her diagnosis had been extremely stressful, involving the suicide of one of her brothers, a move to another country and separation from her husband. The disease gave her a focus around which she was able to make a new commitment to life, to what King calls 'the flow of power and love in the universe', and to transform herself and find peace and healing. 'Leukaemia was the best thing that ever came my way, because I learned much more about myself much more quickly than I ever could have without it.' (Petrea King, 1992)

Spiritually awakened patients may in the end die of the cancer, but nevertheless, they may be grateful – even in the face of self-extinction – that they have woken to a more profound consciousness of existence and of their own lives.

And the curious thing is this: the energy released by this awareness often does put the cancer into remission. It can also make the remaining life more intensely felt and so more profoundly lived. It is also true that this acceptance of illness is one way in which patients can demonstrate that they have accepted themselves. This acceptance can transform your entire subjective world, which in turn can lead to the healing of disease.

A Japanese study into patients who went home to die from cancer and instead got well showed that a complete acceptance of God's will – or the will of fate – was a constant theme through all their stories. We can see what this means in more personal terms when we consider the following words of an AIDS patient: 'I deal with this disease by looking at it as one of the best teachers I've ever had. I treat it with respect. I try to love it. I talk to it. I'll say: "You are safe with me. Do not worry. I do not hate you." ' (Young person with AIDS, quoted by Dr Larry Dossey, 1993)

Sumi Jenner says: 'I am now in my ninth year of living with cancer. At least once a day I think of my lump getting smaller and I talk to it. It is like a barometer in my body: it gets hard and angry when I am doing too much. It is soft and pliant when I am relaxed.'

These are the words of two people who live permanently in the face of death – and yet who have found a measure of peace and acceptance. We should learn from their wisdom.

An A–Z of alternative options

The following is a list of therapies and suggestions which have been put forward by others as effective in the battle with cancer – either as a preventative strategy or as a cure. You may have heard of some, such as homeopathy, while others, like photodynamic therapy, are at the forefront of a new medical technological revolution. Still others, such as radionics, may seem uncomfortably New Age and unduly stretch your credulity. I have deliberately allowed the alphabet to brush them up against each other. One woman's meat is another man's poison. Each of us has to decide which options make personal sense and which don't – and even those that don't make sense today may gain some credibility tomorrow. The point is to open our eyes to the wealth of options there are when it comes to protecting ourselves against cancer – and/or fighting a cancer that has already taken root.

Many of these options can – and perhaps should – be used at the same time. Some doctors will be affronted by such an approach. They may say: 'But if your cancer is cured, you won't know which of the options you chose was responsible.' This could be a problem for the scientist, but it is a matter that need not concern the person with cancer. It presupposes that there is a single effective agent, an assumption that may very well be wrong. Even if it is correct, we cannot know in advance which therapy may be the effective one, and we don't have time to find out when our concern is solely with being cured. A further reason for adopting this strategy is that it is clear that many of these approaches are related to each other, and it may be that they are different ways of harnessing the same curative powers.

When Jonnie Oden discovered she had a malignant breast tumour she knew she wasn't going to have an operation – despite her husband Gary's pleadings. The oncologists they consulted were unanimous – the breast had to be removed. But Jonnie had other plans, and with some initial resistance, Gary eventually came to agree with her. Jonnie started on vitamin and herbal supplements, changed her diet, rubbed bloodroot on the skin nearest the tumour, meditated, did visualisation and hooked herself up to a Rife generator. Her tumour continued to grow, doubling in size over the next six weeks. However, she persevered. Then the 'miracle' occurred. The tumour started to shrink. It is still shrinking at the time of writing. The doctors were so surprised that one even called into question the original diagnosis. Jonnie is a classic case of the 'try everything at once' school of thought, and in her case it is showing every sign of working.

It is up to each reader to decide for her or himself whether these options should be the first and preferred cancer treatment; whether they should be complementary to the standard treatments; or left until mainstream medical treatment has been shown to be ineffective. For myself, I know the answer. If ever I have a cancer, I will be looking to an eclectic mix of many of the following therapies, combined with large doses of vitamin C, Omega 3 oils and dietary changes. I have already made some changes to my way of life as a preventative measure. Let's face it – not getting cancer in the first place is the best way of surviving.

And are these therapies guaranteed to work? Of course not. Everyone is different. There are no statistics, and there have been few – if any – rigorous studies. When there have been studies, their sources have sometimes made the results suspect. That's the problem. Choosing the alternative path to recovery is an act of faith. But then again, so is the decision to have radiation, chemotherapy or surgery. There are no studies that say that surgery is better than a grape diet, and there never will be.

It is valid to approach these therapies on the basis of a risk-benefit analysis. If the risk appears to be low and the potential benefit high, then there is nothing to lose from following a particular course of treatment. Doctors who insist that proof of value must precede the use of any mode of treatment utterly miss the point. As long as there is no proof that a particular therapy is of no value – and negative proofs are harder to arrive at than positive proofs – and as long as there is little or no danger, then any course of action that makes sense should be followed. All that is required is to accept responsibility for yourself.

Acidophilus and other friendly bacteria

Did you know that you have more bacteria than cells in your body? Most of these bacteria are in the gut. They are vital for the breaking down and digesting of food. They also keep other microbial predators at bay – specifically unfriendly bacteria, viruses and fungi. If you have a fungal or inflammatory attack of the urino-genital system, then taking some capsules of Lactobacillus acidophilus should go some way to solving the problem. Athlete's foot is also amenable. There is a healthy balance between bacteria and yeast, but any sign of a yeast attack should be dealt with by taking acidophilus. It has antibiotic properties that keep viruses under control. Polio viruses, for example, cannot survive in the presence of high concentrations of acidophilus. It also helps to maintain tissues in a state of mild acidity, which is healthy.

These bacteria help protect against cancer, and even have an anti-tumour effect. Mice receiving acidophilus supplements showed 400 per cent greater macrophage activity. Macrophages are the blood components that attack cancer tumours. Animal studies show that acidophilus helps to slow down, and even stop, tumour growth.

A Bulgarian doctor, Dr Ivan Bogdanov, using a highly concentrated form of another bacterium, Lactobacillus bulgaricus, obtained a complete remission in a patient suffering from terminal multiple myeloma. The patient was sinking into a coma when treatment started. Six months later, there was no sign of the disease. His only treatment was with the bacteria. In the Bulgarian study, similar results were obtained with people suffering from many types of cancer.

The amounts they took on a daily basis were equivalent to eating 40–60 kg (89–133 lb) of Bulgarian yoghurt. The bacteria-rich product used is called Anabol. The daily dose is 10–15 grams (up to ½ oz). More than this results in the possibility of tumour disintegration, a process which floods the body with toxic products and can kill the patient if detoxification procedures are not started immediately. (For further information, read *Probiotics*, by Leon Chaitow and Natasha Trenev.)

Lactobacillus acidophilus is widely available, but should

221

be kept refrigerated in the shop and at home. Potency of capsules is highly variable, so look around until you get a good supplier.[23]

Acupuncture

The Chinese believe that living energy moves through the body along certain channels, which are sometimes called meridians. This energy, which they call qi (pronounced 'chi'), may become blocked or impeded. It may become sluggish. Through acupuncture, these negative effects may be overcome. No-one claims that acupuncture can cure cancer by itself. Indeed, acupuncturists are very careful to distance themselves from any such claim. However, one British veterinary surgeon, John Carter, has used acupuncture successfully as part of an anti-cancer therapy for animals. His approach is being tested by the Imperial Cancer Research Fund. Results of these tests appear to be promising, but have not yet been released.

Acupuncture can also be effective in helping reduce the side-effects of cancer, or the treatments used to combat it. In Northern Ireland, doctors have used electroacupuncture to relieve the sickness or nausea associated with chemotherapy. The relief, unfortunately, tends to be short-lived. However, with repeated applications, long-term substantial relief can be obtained.

There is some evidence that acupuncture can play a useful role in unblocking the energy flows of the meridians. These meridians, or channels, exist, although they do not correspond to any of the organs. However, various researchers have been able to measure their activity – and it has been found that meridians develop in the pre-formed foetal body before organs do. It is therefore thought that the meridians play an important role in determining the development and alignment of the organs. By freeing the energy flow through these meridians, acupuncture treatment can promote health in the associated organs.

A word of caution: make sure the acupuncturist uses properly sterilised – or new, disposable – needles.

Aromatherapy

In France, aromatherapy is much more accepted than in Britain as a clinically effective therapy for a wide range of chronic illnesses. French doctors often apply it as part of a total treatment plan. Given aromatherapy's short history and the general lack of scientific attention paid to the healing properties of essential oils, and the fact that most British aromatherapists are not doctors (though many are nurses or trained as paramedics), it is not surprising that aromatherapists steer clear of the ethical and legal difficulties that any claim to providing a cancer cure would bring. Nevertheless, there are good reasons why aromatherapy might have a useful part to play.

Firstly, it is well established that a number of oils have an immune system enhancing effect. Secondly, some essential oils are believed to have a broad anti-carcinogenic effect. The following have been proposed by aromatherapist Robert Tisserand as possibly falling into this category: cedarwood, cypress, eucalyptus, hyssop, bergamot and geranium. Thirdly, since stress is a commonly quoted cause of cancer, the calming lavender and energising peppermint oils may also be useful.

Finally, there are those oils that are considered beneficial for the liver, rosemary being one. Since the liver has been implicated by many as the source of cancer, these oils may have a general preventative role to play. The rosemary herb is also considered useful for cancer protection.

Clove oil has been recommended by R. Gattefossé, one of the great French aromatherapists, as having anti-carcinogenic properties. The reasoning is this: cancer cells display reduced cellular magnetic fields. Clove oil has high electrical resistance. When clove oil is taken into these cells, it changes the electro-magnetic properties in the direction of good health.

Patricia Davis, principal of The London School of Aromatherapy, recommends that the oils of garlic, onion, sage and tarragon can also be beneficial. Davis, however, cautions against the use of any aromatherapeutic agent during and for a long time after chemotherapy. This goes against other findings that indicate that cancer patients self-treating with aromatherapy have higher morale. Advice should be taken on this question.

There is also evidence that niaouli or tea tree oil smeared on the skin before radiation may help prevent burning and scarring of the skin. A bath in these oils before treatment may have beneficial effects internally (three to four drops in a full bath). Lavender should be rubbed on after a bath, or bathed in (four to six drops in a full bath). The skin is a highly absorbent organ, and essential oils are very potent, so do not be tempted to exceed five to six drops in total in a bath. Lavender is the great healer and relaxer, so it should be taken in the evening rather than the morning. Peppermint, rosemary and tea tree oil, however, have a bracing quality that makes them ideal for the morning.

Sometimes, a drop of an oil in a glass of water can be drunk, but the other common use for aromatherapy oils is in massage (see Massage, page 273).

Art therapy

With art therapy, as with writing therapy, it is important that the person undergoing the therapy should work without guidance and without judgement on what is produced. The patient should seek to drift into a kind of automatism, or free association, so that material from the unconscious has a chance to rise to the surface.

This type of therapy operates on a number of levels. As a form of creative self-expression, it fulfils a deep inner urge. By establishing contact with the unconscious, the patient finds an outlet for repressed thoughts, wishes and fears. By externalising the sources of conflict, the patient starts a healing process, becoming his or her own therapist. The artistic products can be a source of reference during formal or informal counselling sessions.

The purpose of this therapy is to help the person come to understand him/herself and to be able to confront hidden psychological spectres. In so doing, the chains that tie the ill person to negative emotions, and negative energies, may be released from the body.

Bio-electric therapies

Electrical energy is one of the ultimates of the universe. We are all wrapped in an envelope of electrical-magnetic energy. Even cells generate their own electrical fields. Every activity of the body can be measured electrically. Harold Burr, a Yale University professor, spent several decades studying these electrodynamic fields, or L-fields, as he called them – 'L' for life. Through these L-fields, he believed, we are connected to the entire universe.

This way of looking at the body has been largely ignored by the orthodox medical community until recently, when bio-electrical machines have been introduced to some hospitals to help stimulate tissue repair, especially bone fractures.

Certainly, there are two cautions that need to be made to anyone considering using a bio-electrical approach. The first is that man-made electrical systems tend to have very negative effects on the body. Some evidence suggests that electrical pollution, from pylons for example and electric blankets, can be a cause of cancer. Secondly, electromagnetic treatments that use incorrect polarities may encourage tumour growth rather than retard it. However, there have been a number of interesting and, by all accounts, extremely exciting results from using electromagnetic equipment.

MAGNETS

Some doctors are experimenting with magnets. Dr William Philpott of Choctaw, Oklahoma, treated a twenty-year-old patient with an inoperable glioblastoma – a form of brain cancer. He placed the north pole of a ceramic magnet on the back of the patient's head at the point where the tumour had initially started to grow. The magnet was left in this position for twenty-four hours a day.

At the beginning of the treatment at the American Biologics hospital in Tijuana, Mexico, this patient was incapable of making any response to his environment. After three days of continuous treatment, he was able to wiggle his fingers in response to questions. Three weeks later, he walked out of the hospital with the assistance of only a walking frame. The patient continued magnetic-field exposure of the brain for five hours a day, and was reported to be well six months later except for a residual balance problem.

Obviously, a normal bar magnet is of no use for this kind of treatment, as both north and south poles appear on the same side. What is needed is a flat magnet, magnetised so that opposite poles are on opposing flat sides. (Note that biomagnetic south fields must be avoided. To check the north and south poles of a magnet, you need to use a magnetometer. North pole reads negative, south positive.)

It is also possible to buy magnetic beds to sleep on. Japanese beds are based on normal magnets that have an alternating current force field. These can give temporary benefits, but for long-term benefits a direct current negative field bed is required. One developed by Dr Bronlie, marketed by Magnetico, has a force field nearly ten times stronger than that we currently experience emanating from the earth.

Bronlie's research produced evidence that the magnetic force of the earth is depleting at a rate of five per cent every century – and his bed therefore gives off a magnetic force equal to that prevalent on earth some 4,000 years ago. The flow of this magnetic energy through the body for eight hours a day has had, he claims, a remarkable effect on healing, particularly with arthritis, but more interestingly for our purposes, it has a demonstrable and powerful effect on the oxygen levels in the blood and the efficiency of the body's bio-chemical reactions. Most athletes find it very difficult to improve their VO2 max readings – this is a measure of the maximum amount of oxygen they can use. However, over a matter of months, Canadian athletes lying on his magnetic bed were able to improve this by thirty per cent – an amazing finding. Also, the amount of oxygen in the bloodstream increased. This suggests that the magnetic bed could have a powerful beneficial effect against cancer. But if you buy one, don't take your credit cards into the bedroom!

Bear in mind that this bio-magnetic research is done in the northern hemisphere, where the background magnetic field emanating from the earth is also negative. The earth's magnetic field in the southern hemisphere is the opposite – i.e. positive. For those living below the equator, the magnetic bed manufacturers have a positive bed. The object is to enhance the background radiation, as this enhances the rate of the body's bio-chemical processes. For further information about magnetic beds and other electro-magnetic devices, see Resources.[24]

Many eminent doctors have believed that the body has the properties of a magnet. Franz Mesmer, who died in 1815 and gave his name to mesmerism, treated people in a tub of 'magnetised' water. Harriet Martineau, an English Victorian writer, became a chronic invalid. The best efforts of all the leading doctors did nothing for her. For five years she suffered until, in 1844, a travelling magnetiser named Pencer Hall treated her. His treatment consisted of giving her 'magnetic passes'. After three days, she was able to eat and sleep comfortably for the first time in five years. Thereafter, the treatment was continued by her maid.

It is claimed that individual bio-electric potential can be built up through breathing exercises and meditation.

MICROWAVE RESONANCE THERAPY (MRT)
This is a high-intensity, low-frequency treatment applied to acupuncture points to treat entire acupuncture meridians, so encouraging the body to return to physiological equilibrium – known as homeostasis. It has been developed by Professor Sergei Sitko in Russia. He has used this on over 8,000 patients suffering from a wide range of illnesses.

THE BODY'S OWN ELECTRICAL IMPULSES
For the specific use of electrical impulses to kill a cancer tumour, we can turn to the work of Professor Bjorn Nordstrom, a former head of the Karolinska Institute in Stockholm. He inserts the positive end of a needle electrode into a tumour and places the negative end on the patient's skin. This has resulted in many tumour regressions, and occasionally in a true remission. A single treatment is sufficient for each tumour. It takes one to three hours a session, and can generally be done under local anaesthetic.

Why does this work? Professor Nordstrom believes a number of factors are involved. One is that white blood cells have a slight negative charge, so they will be attracted to a site that is positively charged. Secondly, the electrolysis has a direct tumour killing capability. Nordstrom denies that his electrical stimulation of the sites can have any cancer-causing potential. He makes the point that acute (i.e. high-intensity but short-term) doses of chemicals or electricity do not cause cancer while chronic (long-term) exposure to almost anything may indeed cause cancer – even very low doses of electrical pollution. Since he supplies short-term acute exposure, there is no danger. Chinese doctors are experimenting with this technique with good

227

results. It is also practised in the American Biologics hospital in Tijuana, Mexico. (See also Rife generator and Lakhovsky's cosmic energy cure.)

Borysenko's twelve steps to a healthy life

Joan Borysenko works at a clinic, attached to a major Boston hospital, which has as its aim the harnessing of the mind to help the body fight off disease. She has devised a twelve-step guide to healthy living.

1. Accept that you can't control the external circumstances of your life, but that you can control your responses to them. Reframe your responses so that they lead to positive actions and feelings.
2. Good health depends on both physical and mental factors: so eat properly, exercise properly and meditate regularly.
3. Think of yourself as healthy. Don't think of yourself as unhealthy.
4. Change is the only constant fact of life, so be open to change and absorb change into your life. Don't resist change or complain about it.
5. Your beliefs are more powerful than you know. Become aware of them. Monitor them and make sure they are positive. If they aren't, change them.
6. The only way to escape from stress, fear and doubt is to confront the causes of these emotions directly.
7. The two fundamental emotions are fear and love. Always choose love.
8. When it is a choice between being right or being at peace, choose peace.
9. Accept yourself as you are. Everyone is flawed. Everyone has been hurt. Everyone has had to deal with bitterness. No-one is perfect. We are who we are.
10. When you feel angry or resentful, stop the emotions and practise forgiveness – including forgiveness of yourself.
11. Life never tires of teaching us new lessons. The healthy person is always open to learning and discovering. 'When the student is ready the teacher will appear.'
12. Be patient. Being patient doesn't mean repressing

your impatience, but rather having a mindful attention to the processes around you rather than concern over the speedy realisation of the products of these processes.

To this set of instructions, one more can be added: love and honour yourself.

Breathing

Since stress is a major cause of cancer, it is helpful if we can learn to relax. But breathing exercises are not just stress-busters – they are fundamental to good health and energy. 'How we breathe both reflects the state of the nervous system and influences the state of the nervous system,' says Dr Andrew Weil in his book, *Spontaneous Healing*. He describes five breathing techniques that will lead to improved health and vigour if practised every day.

1. Just observe your inhalations and exhalations for a few minutes. Don't try to influence them. Do this while in a comfortable position, with your eyes closed.
2. Repeat the above, but mentally view the cycle of breath as starting with the exhalation. This actually increases the amount of air inhaled.
3. While seated, or better, while lying down, imagine that the breaths that go out and in do not start with you but originate with the universe itself. You are in the way of the cosmic breath. The universe is breathing itself through you. Feel this universal breath permeating every part of your body.
4. *Stimulating breath*: Sit comfortably with back straight and eyes closed. Place the tip of the tongue on the flesh just above the back of the top teeth: the so-called yogic position. Now breathe in and out rapidly through the nose, keeping the mouth lightly closed. The rhythm of in and out breaths should be rapid, even and audible. Increase duration from fifteen seconds to a minute. This is an energy booster if done regularly, and can be done whenever you feel sleepy and want to keep awake.
5. *Relaxing breath*: This can be done sitting or lying down with the tongue in the yogic position as with the

229

previous exercise. Breathe out with an audible sound, completely emptying the lungs to a count of eight. Then close the mouth and inhale quietly for a count of four. Then hold the breath for a count of seven. Do this for four, building up to eight cycles after a month. Speed is not important, though slow is better than fast.

These breathing exercises are spiritual practices aimed at bringing mind and body to a single focus of energy. Going on from breathing, you can, in the mind's eye, let the breath escape from the nostril and follow it up the nose over the face, follow it as it explores the cheeks, the skull and the locus of nerves at the back of the neck. Let it flow down the arms, down the back, round the buttocks, the legs, the feet, the toes, then back up the leg, the thighs and the pelvic area. Let it rest in the solar plexus for a while, then let it move up over the belly and chest and back up the neck to the nose. While your mind is following this route, let it sift the impressions that arise: was there a twinge or pain anywhere? This is a way of listening to the body.

The quality of breathing has a direct influence on the levels of oxygen in the blood and tissues – which in turn has a direct influence on whether the body's tissues are a good seedbed for the development of cancer tumours.

Brewer's yeast
Normally, healthy people cannot take much brewer's yeast, as it induces nausea. Curiously though, people with cancer have been found to have a very high tolerance for relatively large quantities of this substance – half a cupful a day, or more. This alone may be capable of causing the regression and disappearance of cancers over a one- to three-year period.

A yeast extract is marketed under the name Glucan. In one study, when injected directly into tumours, it caused noticeable shrinkage within ten days.

The Burton approach
Lawrence Burton was not a medical doctor – his doctorate work was in experimental zoology. His specialisation was the relationship between the immune mechanism responses and cancer, first in invertebrates, then in laboratory animals and,

finally, in humans. He graduated in 1955 and for the next eighteen years his life was that of any ordinary highly successful scientist. Eventually he became the senior investigator and oncologist in the cancer research unit of the pathology department of St Vincent's Hospital in New York – a post he held until 1973. It is significant that his cancer research was based in a pathology unit. He was working with real tumours, not cell lines (see page 110), and with real patients, not laboratory rats.

Burton's work led to the development of a serum that would, he argued, inhibit the growth of cancer tumours. This serum was derived from certain proteins found in blood: a tumour antibody, a tumour complement that activates the antibody, an antibody-blocking protein and 'de-blocker' that neutralises the blocker. Burton, with an associate, Frank Friedman, isolated these blood fractions. His theory was that when these four elements were in a balanced ratio in the blood, cancer cells would be routinely destroyed. His serum was a way of bringing about this balance and so putting cancers into remission. Burton called this method of dealing with cancer 'immuno-augmentative therapy'.

The patient's blood is analysed every day to measure the ratio of these four proteins. A personalised serum is then made up to correct any deficiencies in the balance.

Burton's work came to the attention of Pat McGrady, an editor working for the American Cancer Society. McGrady later reported seeing Burton inject some mice with his tumour-inhibiting factor. 'They injected the mice and the lumps went down before your eyes – something I never believed possible.' This demonstration was repeated in 1966 before a group of science writers. The result was a story in the *Los Angeles Times* under the headline: 'Fifteen-minute cancer cure for mice. Humans next'. Oncologists present at the seminar claimed that Burton and Friedman were tricksters.

Eventually, Friedman gave up in disgust and Burton was forced abroad. Despite political interference, the Bahamian government allowed him to set up a clinic in Freeport. There, patients who could afford it made their way to be treated. There were frequent demands from establishment medical bodies for him to conduct clinical trials on his own

– a request he spurned for the obvious reason that, when dealing with the terminally ill, this is tantamount to murder.

In 1985, his clinic was summarily closed down. The National Cancer Institute (NCI) and other bodies had persuaded the Bahamian government that Burton's serum products were a source of hepatitis B and AIDS. The evidence supporting this was of very dubious quality. None of Burton's 2,700 plus patients treated with hundreds of thousands of serum injections ever got AIDS. Impartial experts pointed out, also, that the serum had been put through the wrong test, a test that produces a large number of false positives.

As for hepatitis, only one of Burton's patients came down with this disease. Contrast this with the fact that, in 1976 in the US, blood transfusions caused 30,000 cases of hepatitis, of which 3,000 were fatal. Even before the advent of AIDS, blood transfusions were not a good thing, but the general public have not been kept fully informed of the dangers. According to Dr John Wallace, 'Blood should be regarded as a dangerous drug. There are now more than twenty viruses known to be transmissible by transfusion.'

Outraged patients lobbied the US Congress, with the result that Congress ordered a study of alternative cancer therapies – a point that, in future years, may be seen as the year the tide turned in America in favour of non-orthodox medicine. Dr Burton was allowed to reopen his clinic, which continues the work even though Burton himself died of heart disease in 1993, aged sixty-seven.

Does it work? One patient, Curry Hutchinson, diagnosed as having metastasised malignant melanoma of the lung, told the authors of a *Penthouse* article: 'When I came here I was in a wheelchair. My mother had to care for me constantly. Two months later she was able to go home. I'm walking, jogging, swimming – alive. My improvements are unbelievable. Burton's critics claim there's no proof his therapy works. I disagree. I'm proof.'

See Resources for further information.[25]

The Burzynski method

Dr Stanislaw Burzynski is a doctor and bio-chemist who works in Houston, Texas. His discovery is that a group of peptides and amino acid derivatives occurring naturally in our bodies have the effect of inhibiting the growth of cancer cells. Burzynski calls these peptides antineoplastons.

In Burzynski's view, there is a bio-chemical defence system which allows defective cells to be corrected through bio-chemical means. Antineoplastons are at the heart of this defence system. Blood samples from cancer patients show that they have only two to three per cent of the amount typically found in a healthy person.

Burzynski's method simply requires the injection of anti-neoplastons into the bloodstream. The result is tumour shrinkage, and even remission. Often this occurs in a matter of a few weeks. Burzynski has been treating patients since 1977. He does not claim to be able to cure all cancers in all patients – but there is strong evidence that many are cured. In one study of twenty patients with advanced astrocytoma, a highly malignant brain cancer, four went into early remission, two showed partial remission, and ten showed stabilisation, i.e. tumour regression of less than fifty per cent. Some of these subsequently went on to complete remission.

Burzynski holds more than twenty patents and has had more than 150 papers published. Nevertheless, he is considered a quack by the FDA and the ACS. Some insurance companies refuse to cover his treatments. Antineoplaston was placed in the alternative medicine's hall of fame, the list of 'unproven therapies', in 1983. Even official reports show that Burzynski's treatment has resulted in objective improvements in eighty-six per cent of advanced cancer patients. The FDA took him to court in 1983, and legal action against him has continued. He was allowed to continue his work, but only in the State of Texas – and none of his drugs could be shipped across state lines.

Contact Burzynski's clinic in Texas for details of treatment, and costs. (Treatment can only be conducted at his Texas clinic because of the legal circumstances outlined above.)[26]

CanCell

CanCell is the name given to a substance developed in 1936 by James Sheridan, a chemist working at the time for Dow Chemical, and which was then subsequently taken up and slightly adapted by metallurgist Edward Sopcak in 1984. Sopcak registered the CanCell trademark but he, like Sheridan before him, refuses to sell the substance – it is given away. Both of them claim that 80 per cent of any random group of cancer patients will be cured using CanCell.

The concept underlying CanCell is that the difference between a normal cell and a cancer cell is one of vibrational energy. By manipulating the chemical vibrational frequency of the cell, the cancer cell can be made to self-destruct through a process of self digestion. The resulting material – like raw egg whites – is eliminated by the body any way it can – through urine, stools, vaginal discharge, by coughing and even sweat. CanCell works, therefore, by changing the vibrational frequency of the cell.

There is nothing natural in CanCell. It consists of a number of chemicals chosen for their electrical properties. The formula has never been finalised and is constantly being tinkered with.

Because of the conditions under which CanCell is made available supplies are limited and it must be requested verbally by the person who intends to use it. It is also available for use in AIDS, multiple sclerosis, muscular dystrophy, Parkinson's and Alzheimer's.[27] (See Trull, 1993)

Carnivora

Carnivora is an extract from the digestive juices of the venus fly trap. This plant is very good at digesting animal proteins, and it caught the attention of a German oncologist called Helmut Keller. Dr Keller has tested carnivora on both animals and humans at his clinic in Germany – with good results.

Carnivora contains a powerful chemical, plumbagin, which has demonstrated clear anti-viral and anti-cancer properties in independent tests. It does this by promoting the cellular production of hydrogen peroxide. It is also a powerful healer – yet it is so harmless that the Russians have suggested it can be used as a food preservative.

Self-administered venus fly trap juice is not advised, as it contains other chemicals that can cause unpleasant side-effects. Keller's carnivora has been purified. For further information, see Resources.[28]

Castor oil

The value of castor oil as a healing agent has been known for centuries. It helps to detoxify the liver, and has a direct healing effect on cancerous wounds.

Dr Max Gerson recommended drinking two tablespoons of castor oil each morning followed by a castor oil enema – not a high colonic – five hours later. For surface ulcerating cancer tumours, a flannel cloth should be thoroughly wet with castor oil and placed over the wound. Over this, place a plastic sheet, with an electric heating pad on top. Keep this in place with a towel or bandage. The pack should remain for one to one and a half hours.

Naturopath Jan de Vries comments: 'I recently saw a weeping carcinogenic wound that was cured with the use of a castor oil pack.'

Chelation

Chelation therapy was designed for heart patients. It is a method by which unwanted metals are purged from the system by putting another substance – which binds to the metals and so flushes them out – through that system.

The need for such a chelating substance was strongly felt by industry before the Second World War – the paint, rubber, petroleum and electro-plating industries all needed substances that would bind and eliminate corruption. Research in pre-war Germany came up with an extremely good substance: ethylene-diamine-tetra-acetate, known since then as EDTA. Its first use for medical purposes was in 1947, to clear the bloodstream of a cancer patient suffering toxic side-effects of chemotherapy. It did the trick. In the early 1950s, EDTA was used in a number of circumstances where workers were suffering in large numbers from heavy metal poisoning. In every case, it worked marvellously, according to Harold and Arline Brecher, who have written a number of books on chelation therapy:

> The treated [men] spontaneously reported unanticipated health benefits. Among the varied improvements were increased endurance, improved stamina, better memory, enhanced vision, hearing and smell, clearer thinking, fewer headaches, less anxiety. Those with early signs of arthritis or atherosclerosis enjoyed even more extraordinary recovery – increased mobility, reduced leg cramps, easier breathing.

Since then, hundreds of studies have consistently shown the benefits of chelation therapy, particularly for atherosclerosis – a problem for which the heart bypass operation was designed.

Additionally, it appears that chelation therapy has a possible cancer preventative action. The evidence? A Swiss study investigating the link between lead-based gas fumes and cancer incidence by Drs W. Blumer and T. Reich, based on the health records of 231 Swiss citizens living next to a heavily used highway, showed that cancer mortality among this group was significantly higher than among people living in a traffic-free section of the same town. In both groups, the subjects studied were life-long inhabitants of their respective areas. However, there was a curious exception. One group of the fume-exposed population had developed such severe symptoms of lead poisoning that they had been detoxified with the usual treatment for lead poisoning – EDTA.

As a result, Blumer and Reich were in a position to compare long-term death rates in a matched population of chelated and non-chelated patients. They found a significant mortality difference between the two groups. Of the 231 people in the study, fifty-nine adults had chelation; 172 matched controls did not. Only one (1.7 per cent of the chelated persons) died of cancer, as compared with thirty (seventeen per cent) of the non-treated. After exploring all possible explanations for this statistical disparity in cancer mortality, the authors concluded that chelation was the sole reason for the ninety per cent decrease in cancer deaths.

This supports the experience of doctors who use chelation in their practices. One, Dr E.W. McDonagh, founder member of the International Academy of Preventive Medicine, found that of 25,000 patients that he had treated with chelation, only one of those who had not previously had cancer was later diagnosed as having cancer. Taking this as an indication of chelation's merits, he looked for cases of Vietnam veterans who had been severely poisoned by Agent Orange. This group is known to suffer very high incidences of cancer. He found sixty-three cases who had also, later, had EDTA. Not one of them subsequently developed cancer.

Not all doctors are convinced of this anti-cancer effect. And chelation may not be so effective if cancer had started to develop before the chelation treatment began. 'I have personally seen cancer develop in three people who were undergoing chelation therapy. In these cases, the cancer was present at the start of the chelation, but unrecognised at that time,' according to Dr Harold Steenblock.

How does chelation work, if it does, against cancer? Firstly, by removing toxic metals, it is removing a source of free radicals. It is therefore a preventative measure. For patients who already have cancer, it improves blood circulation by clearing arterial obstructions and so allowing greater supplies of oxygen to reach the cancer site. Cancer tumours do not like high oxygen environments. Also, it is believed that EDTA strips away the protein coat that surrounds tumour cells – this shield is what protects the cancer cells from T-lymphocytes, the white blood cells whose job is to kill invaders. Because of the protein layer, T-lymphocytes do not identify the tumour as an enemy to be overcome. Once this layer has been stripped away, the T-lymphocytes can start to do their job.

During chelation, the patient is hooked up – for two to three hours per session – to an intravenous drip, which contains not only EDTA but also megadoses of vitamins. Increasing numbers of people are undergoing chelation treatments as a general preventative health measure.

A NOTE OF CAUTION
Chelation needs to be carefully administered, as there can be kidney complications from the extraction of too much toxic metal in a short time. A careful graduation of chelation treatments is therefore required. A standard treatment will include around twenty sessions. Also, high supplementation of zinc and selenium is needed, as good metals are taken out with the bad. Some (uncommon) side-effects of chelation may include: low blood calcium, cardiac arrhythmia, fever, headaches and inflammation of the veins. Chelation is contraindicated in the cases of damaged kidneys, liver disease, TB, brain tumours and pregnancy.

See Resources for more information.[29]

Chewing food slowly
This is a key tenet of the macrobiotic approach to health. The thinking behind it is very simple. Firstly, the body

has two basic modes: tense and relaxed. For most people, the body is in a state of more or less constant tension. When the body is tense, adrenaline is released, which triggers the fight or flight response. In this mode, the body is not prepared to absorb all the nutrients in the food. Rather, it is ready for only partial digestion and speedy elimination of the food. Even the food that is digested is not made use of, because the body's cells have other priorities. A relaxed body, however, is able to benefit from the nutrients taken in. Slow chewing will help to relax the body and harmonise the mind.

Additionally, chewing food until it is completely dissolved allows the powerful digestive enzymes in the mouth to predigest the food before it hits the stomach. This allows much better absorption of nutrients. One last benefit of slow chewing is that the body becomes aware of how full it is in time to have an impact on the amount of food eaten.

Coley's toxins

One highly successful method of curing cancer has remained more or less sidelined for over a century. Dr William Coley discovered accidentally that a man had undergone what seemed like a spontaneous remission after suffering from a particular bacterial infection. The toxins that he developed and tested on other patients, often successfully, were the by-products of two bacteria – Streptococcus pyogenes and Serratia marcescens.

The toxins cause a transient but marked fever, accompanied by chills and tremblings. A survey of 1,000 of Coley's cases showed a forty-five to fifty per cent five-year survival rate. The best results were with giant cell bone tumours, where the five-year survival rate was more than eighty per cent. Amazingly, they were then put on the list of unproven treatments by the American Cancer Society (ACS).

Recently, there has been renewed interest in these toxins in China and Germany. A special hospital has been established in Beijing, where cancer patients can be treated with Coley's toxins. In Göttingen, these toxins – under the name of Pyrogenic Bacterial Lysate – have been used in cases of advanced malignant melanoma, which is normally quickly fatal. In three cases out of fifteen,

238

long-term remission was achieved.
See Resources for information.[30]

Colour therapy

This therapy involves irradiating the body – or specific parts of the body – with light of a particular designated colour, which is determined by the therapist after diagnosis of the problem. Colours are forms of electromagnetic radiation, and they inhabit a very narrow stretch of the spectrum of electromagnetic radiation. But just as micro-waves, X-rays and ultra-violet rays have an effect on the body, so too, it is argued, do the different colours – both combined in the form of full-spectrum white light, or separately.

Research has shown that the average light bulb and neon strip, such as provide the lighting in most homes and offices, are not healthy, as they do not provide full-spectrum white light. John Ott, one of the pioneers in the field of light and its effects on health, discovered that full-spectrum lighting helped reduce hyperactivity among children. It was his view that conventional lighting and televisions that leak radiation can cause hyperactivity. The beneficial effects of sunlight are dealt with separately. Here we will look at how colour therapy works.

The colour therapist works with a projector which has five coloured plates – red, yellow, green, blue, violet – that can be used separately or in combination to produce any of the following colours: the primary light colours: red, green and violet; the secondary light colours: yellow, blue and magenta; and the tertiary colours: lemon, orange, turquoise, indigo, purple and scarlet.

Green is the colour that harmonises and maintains the natural physical balance, so this is the colour most often used. Disease and illness cause the body to shift to one side or the other. If it moves more to the yellow, this means the body will be feverish or inflamed. This needs to be corrected with a dose of blue light. If the movement is the other way, towards the blue, then the patient will feel dull and sedated and may need a dose of yellow light.

Each colour has a range of qualities and effects on the body. Red, for example, stimulates the liver and helps build haemoglobin; green stimulates the pituitary and acts as a general purifier and disinfectant; scarlet is aphrodisiac, and stimulates the kidneys; orange is for those with weak lungs and who need to stimulate the thyroid. The colours are light, as opposed to pigment, colours. A course of colour therapy treatments may consist of only four to six sessions.

Colour therapists make two further claims that are less easily accepted. The first is that water poured into a glass of the correct colour will become energised with the qualities of the colour, and can then be drunk as medicine. Secondly, the colour need not be applied directly on the individual's body. In fact, the person can be absent, as long as a 'witness' – such as a drop of blood, a piece of hair or even the person's own handwritten name and address on an envelope – of the patient's presence is used to receive the treatment. An explanation of these claims is given below under Vibrational medicine.

What is it like to receive colour therapy? One patient described her feelings during a session. First the therapist bathed her in a lemon colour. 'At first I felt nothing, but as time progressed there was a feeling of fullness and tightness in the area. By the end, I was feeling just slightly nauseous.' Then the therapist changed the light to a dark red filter. 'I was immediately relieved of the slight discomforts and became aware of a new sensation farther down, a fullness and yet somehow a relaxing and soothing vibration [and after fifteen minutes] I was on the verge of being asleep.' The therapist changed the coloured light to green. 'The moment he did, I was wide awake. My whole body started to tingle. My breath came fast and my heart was pounding. It was most similar to the excitement that builds up just before orgasm.'

In subsequent treatments, this women did not respond so strongly to the sensations, calling them mild. This woman was, it is claimed, cured of fibroids and cancer.

See Resources for further details.[31]

Denial

Twenty years ago, when the impact of personality and attitude on the course of disease first began to gain recognition, it was a given that it was good to face the threat, confront it rationally and take responsible steps to deal with it. Denial and avoidance were wrong. Now the

240

tide has changed. It is recognised that a refusal to face the facts may itself be a health-promoting strategy. If the mind refuses to accept that it has a disease, many of the body's processes will continue on the assumption that there is no disease – which can keep people alive for longer.

Dr Larry Dossey quotes the case of a woman who came to his surgery with an advanced, ulcerating cancer 'as large as a grapefruit' that had spread to her lymph nodes and neck. She told him she had had the tumour for fifteen years. In his view this was impossible, but the woman insisted it was true and her family corroborated this. Her fears that surgery would cause the tumour to run wild proved correct, and she died shortly after her operation.

DMSO (Dimethyl sulphoxide)
DMSO is an organic sulphur compound. It is a clear, colourless and largely odourless liquid that has demonstrated definite anti-tumour qualities. Over 6,000 articles in the scientific literature establish a very solid claim for it to be recognised as an anti-cancer weapon. Vets use it freely when treating cancer in animals. It is available on prescription.

DMSO can be taken by intravenous injection, orally, or it can be rubbed on. It is absorbed very rapidly through the skin, so this is a very efficient way of getting it to the intended site. Patients who wish to undergo radiation and chemotherapy should take DMSO as it also has pain relief abilities and reduces the side-effects of these treatments.

DMSO has a wide range of biological activities. One reason given for this is that it creates very powerful bonds with water molecules. This allows it to penetrate membranes and to pass from one organ, or tissue, to another with great ease. It has a wider range of bio-chemical actions than any other known chemical agent. One Chilean study showed that DMSO, in conjunction with low doses of a chemotherapeutic drug, was able to obtain remissions in forty-four out of sixty-five cancer patients. This result was even more extraordinary, because these patients had all previously had chemotherapy without success. Twenty-six of the cases involved women with metastatic breast cancer. Twenty-three obtained remission. Whether the remission was permanent is not known. It is also not known what

241

effect DMSO on its own, without the chemotherapy, would have had.

There is a theory, rejected by mainstream science, that bacteria known as dwarf bacteria are implicated in some cancers. These bacteria, it is believed, have the ability to change their shape and size and to become as small as a virus. There is experimental support for this suggestion. DMSO, in very low concentrations, has the ability to kill these bacteria. This is impressive, because these bacteria are otherwise extremely drug resistant. DMSO, in a 12.5 per cent solution, shows long-term growth inhibitory action on cancer tumours in laboratory settings.

One dramatic case of a DMSO implicated cancer cure occurred in 1970, when the mother of three-year-old Clyde Robert Lindsey of Pasadena, Texas, took her son to see Dr Eli Tucker of Houston. Clyde had a very deadly cancer, known as Letterer-Siwe disease. The cancer had spread throughout his body, and orthodox doctors considered the case to be hopeless. Dr Tucker gave the boy a dilute mixture of DMSO mixed with haematoxylon, a chemical normally used as a dye to trace the location of pathological animal cells. The haematoxylon-DMSO combination therefore had a special affinity for tumour cells. Inside the cells, the haematoxylon oxidises, with the effect of inactivating the substance that surrounds the cancer cells, which then starve to death. Five drops of this substance in a glass of distilled water every morning from then until now eliminated Clyde's cancer – and he is still alive today.

SIDE-EFFECTS – AND A CAUTION
Side-effects may include a garlicky taste in the mouth and bad smell on the breath. Some people suffer from headaches, dizziness and mild nausea. A localised skin rash or burning feeling can occur on the skin.

Anyone using DMSO should use only 99.9 per cent pharmaceutical grade. All jewellery should be removed before use, and care needs to be taken that the DMSO does not come into contact with clothing. It is a powerful solvent. Care also needs to be taken to ensure that no contamination occurs, as otherwise potentially toxic substances may be absorbed into the body along with the

DMSO. This characteristic can be used to good effect, as the DMSO can – as well as having its own anti-carcinogenic effect – take other substances, such as vitamin C, deep into the body.

To test for purity of DMSO, put the bottle in the fridge, not the freezer. Pure DMSO crystallises at 68°F (20°C) – if it doesn't crystallise, it is not pure. When purchasing it, state that the DMSO is required to be used as a solvent – it cannot be sold for cancer treatment.

For a partial listing of centres offering DMSO therapy, see *Third Opinion: An International Directory to Alternative Therapy Centers for the Treatment and Prevention of Cancer* by John Fink. See Resources for sources of DMSO.[32]

Embracing nature

Just as some people are more eccentric than others, so too do some therapies appear more eccentric. This is true of those who favour embracing the earth or the trees that grow. My feeling is that if these therapies have value – and why should they not? – it may be in some way related to the vibrational medicine discussed below.

Francis Bacon, the seventeenth-century writer and philosopher, described the value of nature's embrace: 'I knew a man that lived long, who had a clean clod of earth brought to him every morning as he sat in bed, and he would hold his head over it a good long while.' Following a plough was considered invigorating. Some believe that a man can recharge his energies by walking barefoot on natural soil, grass or sand.

Tree hugging is also believed to be health promoting. The living energy of the tree strengthens the living energy that flows through us. So, go hug a tree! Lakhovsky went further, believing that people who ate vegetables and fruit grown in their own garden and drank well water from their own locality were strongly protected against cancer. A full account of his theories appears in his book *The Secret of Life*.

Exercise

Studies have shown that a one- to two-mile walk three or four times a week helps enormously in stabilising the disease progress – and sometimes reversing it. A walk like this helps the appetite, sleep cycle and energy level. Exercise is always helpful and immune enhancing – as long as you don't go past the point of being tired, and allow sufficient time for recovery between sessions.

How can exercise help? By increasing the blood's oxygen levels and so decreasing the qualities in the body that make it an easy place for a cancer tumour to live.

Chinese qigong exercises have been implicated in some cancer success stories. As with all Chinese martial arts, they require controlled, deep breathing rhythms. The qigong exercises are specifically designed to promote good breathing habits.

Dr Maude Tresillian Fere's cure

Dr Maude Tresillian Fere cured herself of bowel cancer without the aid of surgery, radiation or chemotherapy. She objected profoundly to the latter methods of dealing with cancer, although she was in every other way an orthodox doctor. It was her view that cancer was caused by an excess of sodium in the system. Since this was a whole-body problem, a part-body solution could not be successful.

Dr Fere's treatment consisted of the following:

1. Ammonium chloride: one 7.5 grain tablet three times daily, half an hour before meals.
2. Liquid diluted phosphoric acid: in the proportion of one teaspoonful in two tablespoons water, half an hour after each meal.
3. Tincture of iodine: one teaspoon of iodine tincture to 10 grams water. One teaspoon a day, at any time.
4. 'Acidulated water': standard strength dilute hydrochloric acid: dilute one teaspoon in a pint and a quarter of cold boiled water. Drink half mid-morning, half mid-afternoon.
5. 'Stock vinegar': one tablespoon of standard strength diluted hydrochloric acid in half a pint of cold boiled water. A teaspoon of this mixture to be taken with a quarter pint of milk once a day. Plastic spoons should be used. (This can be taken with carrot juice as a replacement for the acidulated water.)
6. A strictly vegetarian diet for three months, with fresh

vegetables very lightly cooked, with nuts and sweet fruits like raisins, dates, etc.
7. No bottled, tinned or preserved foods, no salt of any kind – salt-free butter, bread, etc. – sugar, tea, coffee, alcohol, condiments or spices.

It took Dr Fere two years before she felt she had been fully cured. This regime must be followed without deviation. But as a doctor, she has a low regard for the average patient's discipline: 'In dealing with any case of serious illness, I have always tried to enlist the assistance of a person other than the patient to act as a guarantor that the instructions are carried out exactly.' She did not trust even herself, and found someone else to make sure she kept to her regime.

Analysing her treatment, we can see that she mixed two concepts – that of maintaining a low sodium, high potassium balance, and ensuring the right pH balance. For further information about her approach to diet and cancer, see Fere's book, *Does Diet Cure Cancer?*.

Fever therapy

One ancient Greek doctor said: 'Give me the power to produce fever and I'll cure all disease.' Fever, of course, is not a disease in itself, but is a symptom that the body is fighting off some disease. It is generally a very effective defence. Many invading bodies die when the body's temperature rises. Fever promotes the body's own defence mechanisms – detoxifying enzymes and white blood cells are released into the system in higher concentrations. Therefore, fevers should be encouraged, not artificially cooled down. Fever therapy is simply the harnessing of this knowledge for the purposes of inducing high fever under clinical conditions.

An active fever can be induced by the injection of the drug vaccincurin, or pyrifer. A passive fever can be induced by placing the patient inside a cylinder and subjecting him or her to ultra-short waves. Modern medicine has developed other ways of interfering with the thermostats in the brain. They can even raise the temperature of selected portions of the body without affecting other parts. The object is to bring the patient to a state where his body temperature is

105–108°F (40–42°C) for between one and one and a half hours, the temperature at which cancer cells are damaged, but not normal cells. During this treatment, the body loses potassium, so a potassium-rich diet must be maintained: lots of bananas, rice and potatoes. Healthy cells are not damaged until temperatures rise to 109.5°F (43°C). Sometimes heat can be applied to a solid tumour through a heat probe placed inside the lump.

This therapy can even be done at home. The patient can sit in a very hot bath and then lie in bed surrounded by blankets and hot water bottles for five or six hours at a time. Passive fever treatments are usually done three times a week, for as long as it takes. Fever can also be produced by hypnotic suggestion. Some doctors use this therapy in conjunction with chemotherapy – allowing them to lower doses by a third or even a half.

Syphilis was cured by fever therapy before the discovery of penicillin. The means by which the cure was effected was to infect the syphilitic patient with malaria. The result? Regular and persistent fevers that took the body's temperature to 104°F or 105°F (40°C) for the necessary duration. Then the malaria could be cured with quinine. For this line of reasoning, Professor Julius Wagner von Jauregg won the Nobel Prize in 1927.

Flower therapy

It is part of common folklore that some people have green fingers – they appear to have a special affinity with plants, and plants respond to their touch. 'All flowers talk to me, and I reply,' said the chemist, George Washington Carver. Some people claim that simply by directing loving thoughts, they can positively influence the growth of plants.

One person who had such an affinity was Edward Bach, a Welsh doctor who gave up his practice to develop a healing system based on flower essences. He extracted them by steeping the flowers in spring water in the sunlight. The purpose of these essences is to direct our individual spiritual, emotional, mental and physical development in the direction of health. According to Dr Bach: '[Disease] is the means adopted by our own souls to point out to us our faults, to prevent our making greater errors, to hinder us from doing more harm, and to bring us back to the path of Truth and Light from which we should never have strayed.'

For Dr Bach, disease does not have a physical cause, but is the result of a spiritual disharmony within the person. It was his belief that each individual has a spiritual dimension, which is the soul. This soul is aware of the individual's life mission, which needs to be given expression in his or her physical, mental and emotional life. But when a person deviates from the mission, or is blind, deaf and unfeeling to the promptings of the true mission, the result is disease. The worst of all the errors is when love is not freed, but is instead denied.

Disharmony results in various negative emotional states. By correcting these states, harmony can be restored. Flower essences work, it is argued, by radiating harmonious energy at frequencies that help to correct distortions in the energy field of the patient. The idea has been developed in Australia and the US, so it is now possible to choose from a range of over one hundred essences.

One way of choosing which Bach flower essence to use is simply to sniff each of the thirty-eight essences that Edward Bach found and to see which of them the mind and body respond to. Another way is to read the list of emotional states that they are good for dealing with. A number of different 'remedies' can be taken at the same time, up to a maximum of six. For emergencies, and particularly for anxiety attacks, a ready-mixed Rescue Remedy is available.

For the cancer patient who is self-denying, the following remedies may be useful: agrimony, centaury, chicory and red chestnut. For those who are overly strict and rigid: rock water. Violet gives feelings of placidity, gentian dissipates depression. For those feeling depression, desperation or despair, any of the following may be helpful: larch, pine, elm, sweet chestnut, star of Bethlehem, willow, oak or crab apple. For those undergoing recovery from traumatic events: walnut and willow. Three to five drops are taken four times a day, with or without water.

Bach flower remedies are widely available in health shops.

Group support
There is strong evidence that those who live within a

247

network of strong social relationships live longer and healthier lives. Loneliness kills. Group support heals. Women who attend support groups, for example, do much better than women who do not. Some studies have shown that women having regular group therapy live twice as long as those who don't.

Almost every new cancer patient is faced with the problem of who to tell and what to say about the disease. Some people bottle it up and keep it to themselves. Generally speaking, this is not a good idea, as it prevents others from giving support or providing information that may be helpful. The best strategy is to tell everyone everything. It really does get a lot of nonsense out of the way.

If group therapy is desired, your doctor should be able to point you in the right direction. However, take care to find the right kind of support group. A group of women who have all had mastectomies, for example, would be very good support for any new member who had also had a mastectomy – but not necessarily for a woman who had refused a mastectomy. It depends on the group's attitude. If they support her plan, that's good. If they try to get the woman in question to get used to the idea of the necessity of mastectomy, then she needs to find another group – fast.

The emphasis of group support should be on helping people to live as fully as possible, to help communication with family members and friends, to help ease the fears of death and dying and to help, where desired, with the release of emotion. One possibly negative feature of group therapy, however, is that it may gradually accustom members to the idea of dying and so place imperceptible obstacles in the way of seeking a cure.

Annette Crisswell, herself a cancer survivor who has facilitated a support group for seven years, provided me with the following guidelines on the subject.

It has been found that people attending a support group do far better in terms of recovery than those who choose not to. However, not everyone flourishes in groups and I believe it is important that they are not made to feel that their chances of recovery are in any way impeded by going it alone. Each person must find

248

the best way back to 'wellness' for themselves, with confidence.

WHAT IS A SUPPORT GROUP?

1. A gathering of people who have experienced a trauma of some kind, such as a life-threatening illness, a traumatic loss, etc. – an experience which has created chaos in their lives.
2. The group may or may not be run by an experienced counsellor. With a counsellor, the group may be based more on group therapy, otherwise a support group is exactly what it says: a group that gives support. It is not there to advise people what they should do, condemn what they have done or to criticise or change how they are.

The purposes of a support group are:

1. To provide information about the various and the latest treatments – allopathic, complementary, alternative – that are available and relevant to the objects of the group; a source of books, articles, etc.
2. To provide a safe place for people to discuss their feelings and fears with those who have, or have had similar experiences, without criticism or negation.
3. To empower people and to revitalise their self-belief.
4. To provide specialist speakers who are able to clarify and give information about different treatments, so that people in the group are able to make informed choices and have their misunderstandings and doubts clarified.

Depending on the needs and desires of its members, a support group can:

1. Be simply a group of people who get together at regular intervals to chat, exchange information, become friends.
2. Be a regular gathering of people for the purpose of experiencing complementary therapies aimed at empowering the body, mind and spirit. This may include counselling sessions. The underlying principle

will be a concern for the whole person of each member of the group.

3. Be a structured series of meetings, say once a week for ten weeks, in which different specialists or practitioners can be invited to give a talk. This can be combined with counselling and group sharing sessions.

4. Organise themselves – as often, but by no means always, happens with cancer support groups – round the different cancers that the individual members have, e.g. breast cancer group, lung cancer group, etc.

The basic rule of any such group is to empower people so that each person is helped to define for him/herself positive action and attitude goals.

It is also important to discuss what a support group is *not*. It is not there to advise anyone on the right thing to do. What is right for one person is not necessarily right for another. Whatever someone chooses to do is right for them and they should be supported in their choice and empowered to realise their chosen goals. Nor is a support group there to counsel people, unless there is an experienced, trained counsellor present.

Too often, empowering people is seen simply as telling people to 'be positive', and in this way attempting to negate fear, anger and sadness. I challenge anyone who has been told that they are going to have a double mastectomy to feel cheerful and positive. Being positive does not mean blinding yourself to all the negative aspects inherent in the situation. In its proper and helpful sense, it is having an attitude that recognises the feelings of sadness and inadequacy, the fears and terrors and all the other complex emotions that are commonly experienced. At the same time, there is an awareness of the options and alternatives – that the future ultimately is not hopeless, that it is not meaningless, that recovery is not impossible, that change for the better will come in its own time and the burdens of the present must be borne until that better time arrives.

People who have attended a support group often say things like: 'I felt so alone until I joined the group. People who have not had this experience just do not understand.' 'It was such a relief to know that how I was reacting was quite normal.' 'It's good to be able to meet people who have been through what I'm going through and have recovered. There is life after cancer.'

Healing sounds

Primal sound therapy, as taught by Deepak Chopra[40] and the Maharishi Ayurveda Health Centres, is based on the idea that all matters of health originate at the 'quantum level' of the body, which is in tune with the energy web of the universe. Ill-health comes when this energy connection is blocked for some reason. It is therefore necessary to open up the energy channels so that we can get back in touch with the primal energy vibrations, which always work in the direction of health. One method of achieving this is to use vibrating sound.

There are a number of sound therapies. Perhaps the simplest to access is that put forward by Jonathan Goldman in this book, *Healing Sounds*. He suggests that an harmonic meditation heals by balancing the chakras. To do this is simple. Place yourself in a comfortable meditation pose and breathe from the abdomen. Then focus on each of the seven chakras in turn, starting from one, the base of the spine (close to the anus); two, a point a few centimetres below the navel; three, the navel; four, the heart (this point is in the centre of the chest, between the nipples); five, the throat; six, the brow, the position of the third eye; seven, the crown, the top of the head. While focusing on each point, make an open-throated vowel humming sound as full of vibrations as is possible, starting with a low tone and an 'uh' or 'ooo' sound. At each chakra point, the tone should shift up a notch and the vowel sound should change like this: uh-ooo-oh-ah-eye-ih-eee.

Jonathan Goldman also claims that healers can use sounds to heal their patients[33].

High and low pH therapies

pH is the standard measure of the acid-alkali levels of any chemical substance. Levels below pH7 are acidic, and levels above pH7 are alkali. In a state of good health, the body has a pH value of 7.4. This balance is determined almost entirely by the foods we eat. Cancer cells show slight acidity, and they produce acidic toxic wastes. The theory behind high pH therapy is that the acidic cancer cells should be neutralised by making the blood slightly alkali.

According to proponents of this therapy, it is therefore important both for cancer prevention and treatment to shift the whole body back to a weakly alkaline state. To achieve this high pH goal, you should take supplements of rubidium carbonate, caesium chloride, caesium carbonate, zinc gluconate, selenium, magnesium, vitamin C and vitamin A. Potassium supplements can also be added, but taken separately from the caesium supplements. When 1 mg of rubidium carbonate was given to mice, they responded well, tumours only growing at less than ten per cent the rate of the controls. This suggests a human dose of 200–400 mg.

In a trial using caesium chloride over three years with a group of fifty terminal cancer cases, twenty-four per cent died in the first two weeks of the trial and another twenty-six per cent died within a year. The remaining fifty per cent, however, showed long-term improvement. Remember, this was with terminal cases who were all expected to die within months, not years. A high level of pain relief was another plus of this treatment, which was felt by all the patients in the study.

Caesium is also reasonably non-toxic and any toxicity it may have can be reduced by taking alcohol.

The ultimate objective of high pH therapy is to achieve a balance of pH8. At this pH level, cell division reportedly stops. However, there is also a contrary approach that seeks to attain a mildly acidic tissue state, i.e. a low pH state. The reasoning behind this therapy is that cells placed in normal sea water will divide at a normal rate, but if even very small amounts of alkaline sodium chloride – table salt – are added to the solution, then the cell multiplication rate increases. This is why table salt has to be completely avoided by cancer patients. If, instead, a mildly acidic substance is added, the cells stop multiplying. 'It is well known that there is an increased alkilinity of the plasma of the blood and body serum in cancer, especially in the fluid surrounding a cancerous tumour. This is exactly what one would expect in a body that has an abnormal amount of sodium.' (Dr Fere, 1963)

Therefore, frequent mild doses of very dilute hydrochloric acid and phosphoric acid are recommended, both of which are present in the normal human body but in short supply in cancer patients.

Apple cider vinegar, diluted in distilled or pure spring water, is very helpful in maintaining a healthy pH tissue level and is, incidentally, both pleasant to drink and a great thirst quencher.

All processed foods are sodium saturated, and should therefore be avoided. If a high sodium intake is necessary, it must be balanced by phosphorus, as this helps to neutralise excess sodium. A standard dilution of phosphoric acid mixed with water, taken after every meal, can help. Phosphorus is also available in raw fruits and vegetables. Anyone taking no salt should ensure that there is a source of iodine in the diet. Dr Gerson recommended half-strength Lugol's solution – a combination of five per cent iodine and ten per cent potassium iodide in water. Iodine invades cancer cells when they are inflamed and inhibits cancer growth.

Homeopathy

The 1994 edition of *Everyone's Guide to Cancer Therapy* says this of homeopathy: 'Around 1850, homeopathy became popular. This was based on its Law of Similia or Similars, which states that disease results from suppressed itch ("Psora"). Over 3,000 drugs, each a highly distilled organic or inorganic substance, were used for cures.' This rather bizarre description does three things very effectively. It says first of all that this is a weird and wonderful, delusionary system of treatment; secondly, it gives the distinct impression that it is based on some arcane and difficult system of belief; and thirdly, the use of the past tense suggests that homeopathy no longer exists.

Homeopathy as a system of treatment is in fact alive and well in many countries throughout the world. It has the blessing of the British royal family – Her Majesty Queen Elizabeth, The Queen Mother, is the patron of the British Homeopathic Association. As she is, at the time of writing, in her late nineties and generally healthy, we should perhaps have respect for whatever medical and dietary regime she is on.

In the UK, it is possible to get homeopathic treatment on the National Health system. There are six homeopathic hospitals in Britain, the largest of which is the Royal

London Homeopathic Hospital in Great Ormond Street. Nevertheless, even in the UK, homeopathy is still viewed with great suspicion by large sections of the medical profession. In 1986, the British Medical Association (BMA) published a report entitled *Alternative Therapy*. In this report, the authors stated their commitment to scientific method in these words: 'Scientific method lays emphasis on observation, measurement and reproducibility.' The report went on to say: 'It is simply not possible, for example, for orthodox scientists to accept that a medicine so dilute that it may contain not so much as one molecule of the remedy in a given dose can have any pharmacological action.'

The kind of medicine being described is homeopathy, and it is being rejected not on the scientific grounds of observation, measurement or reproducibility – but on the ideological grounds that conventional medics cannot understand it. Indeed, the BMA goes on to state that homeopathy is not 'consistent with natural laws as we now understand them'. There is no suggestion that the problem may be with their understanding of natural laws!

A proper scientific approach based on observation, measurement and reproducibility would approach the question differently. A true scientist would say: 'I don't understand how this works, but let's observe and measure and see whether it does in fact have reproducible results.' That would be the proper scientific approach. It is clear that the BMA in 1986 did not enshrine a value-free, scientific approach to medicine.

However, in 1993, a new report was published which took a much more neutral, balanced – even tolerant – stance on the position of alternative therapies. Its purpose was to lay down conditions by which they could enter the umbrella of respected medical therapies. This is a major leap, and a very positive sign that the growing groundswell of opinion is moving the BMA down the right road.

Homeopathy does in fact have a very clear theory – one which is also shared in certain circumstances by orthodox medicine – and one for which there is scientific support. Homeopathy was developed by Samuel Hahnemann as a result of his studies into the effects of quinine. Hahnemann discovered that quinine, in a normally healthy person, creates the same symptoms as malaria. Since it was also a very effective cure for malaria, Hahnemann came to the view that symptoms did not arise from the disease – instead they arose from the body's attempts to fight the disease. So, by exaggerating the symptoms, the disease can be more successfully fought off.

Applied to other areas, this perception has interesting corollaries. A cough should not be suppressed – rather, it should be encouraged. After all, it arises because the body is seeking to expel something. We should help it, because otherwise whatever is causing the irritation will remain in the body. Similarly, a fever should be promoted rather than cooled; the heat of the body is fighting the infection, so we should encourage it to stay hot and so help it defeat the infection sooner. This is a perfectly legitimate – and indeed commonly accepted – point of view, even among some orthodox doctors. Hahnemann followed this logic through to its inevitable conclusion, and suggested that we should use medicines that promote the same symptoms as the disease – the real explanation of his Law of Similars. This is a perfectly simple and reasonable theory, and it goes against no laws of nature.

Hahnemann made the following observation: 'Most medicines have more than one action: the first a direct action, which gradually changes into the second (which I call indirect secondary action). The latter is generally a state exactly the opposite of the former.' We have discovered this effect in chemotherapy – it is known as resistance. A drug attacks the flawed action of the body, i.e. the disease which is embedded in the cells of the body. The cells have a natural tendency to resist this action, so they amplify the original effect. Eventually, the drug's effects are neutralised. The doctor sees that the drug no longer has an effect and withdraws it, with the result that the problem is much worse. Sometimes, of course, the drug is able to so overcome the cells' flawed action that a cure is effected. The problem is in those cases where the drug is not effective. Its effects ultimately are to worsen the problem. Hahnemann therefore had the idea of reversing the process. If you reverse the action by amplifying the effect, the cells will resist this by diminishing the cause – and so working towards a cure. When the drug is

255

removed, the cells are working in the direction of health.

Hahnemann discovered that dilute doses of drugs work better than strong doses. Now, there is nothing in homeopathic theory that predicts this effect. It is the result of an observation. It is therefore the product of value-free science. It is true simply because it has been demonstrated to be true. *Why* it is true is not yet known. Hahnemann experimented with increasingly dilute solutions as he wished to interfere as little as possible with the healing power of the body.

CAN HOMEOPATHY HELP IN THE FIGHT AGAINST CANCER?

Enid Segall, secretary-general of the British Homeopathic Association argues that it can: 'Homeopathy is very supportive to patients with cancer. Certainly, there are people I talk to regularly who have been cured of cancer with the help of homeopathy.'

Homeopathy is a whole-person approach to treatment. It deals with the disease process, rather than the disease product. This distinction remains, as we have seen, the great dividing line between alternative/complementary approaches and the orthodox approach. Homeopaths ask how it is the cancer formed, and what in the body's physical ecology is supporting the cancer's growth. In this, they are in agreement with naturopaths and, indeed, with almost every other practitioner of non-orthodox healing. Most homeopaths recognise that removal of the end product – the cancerous tumour – may be a useful adjunct to their treatment. However, toxic chemotherapy is not one of the forms of treatment they approve of.

Homeopathic treatment is generally proposed as a therapy that supports other therapies. It is believed to be beneficial no matter what other therapies are being used – even in the case of chemotherapy and radiation. It can benefit the patient by reducing side-effects and improving the sense of well-being. Indeed, homeopaths are very cautious about their role in cancer treatment. There seems to be some resistance to the idea that homeopathy alone would be effective in curing cancer, although they would not deny it was possible. Any patient going to a homeopathic hospital with the intention of having homeopathic treatment alone is carefully counselled and reminded that

256

there are limitations to this approach.

This generally defensive attitude to homeopathy is a modern phenomenon. One hundred years ago, J. Compton Burnett wrote a short book entitled *The Curability of Tumours by Medicines*. He gives a number of examples of cancer cases that he cured entirely by homeopathic means. The following is a case of breast cancer he describes successfully treating:

> [Jessie S] came on May 24th 1888 and informed me that two years previously a lump came in her left breast, which lump persists in growing, and pains. In the left mamma there was a tumour in its outer lower fourth, about the size of a lady's fist. In three months, the tumour was gone and thus far has not returned. *Thuja* 30, *Acid nit*. 30 and *Sabina* 30 were used in infrequent dose, and each given during one month by itself alone and in order named. I ought to have added to the foregoing narrative that I forbade salt and milk, other than in very moderate quantities, and recommended a partial exclusion of meat from the patient's dietary, as also the ovary irritating condiment known as pepper. Pepper, salt and milk are bad in cases of mammary tumours from ovarian or uterine irritation, and many of these tumours are of such origin.

Salt and milk have been widely implicated as nutritional no-nos, but pepper? Modern science comes to Dr Compton Burnett's support. In 1980, researchers found that mice exposed to black pepper developed significantly more tumours – mainly liver, lung and skin. Seventy-seven per cent of the pepper-treated mice developed tumours, compared with only eleven per cent of the controls.

Compton Burnett agrees that it is vital for the homeopathic doctor treating cases of cancer to have the full range of orthodox medical training to help the diagnosis of the ailments. We don't know how many cancer cases Compton Burnett failed to cure, but he certainly felt that his success rate was better than anyone else's – and certainly justified greater attention being given to this medicinal approach to cancer treatment.

Further information can be obtained from Resources.[34]

Hydrazine sulphate

Cancer kills people mainly through causing weight loss and debilitation, a process known to doctors as cachexia. Dr Joseph Gold decided that one way to approach the cancer question was to interfere with cachexia. If he could do this, then although cancer tumours might grow, they wouldn't generally speaking kill the person who had them. Cancer might then be seen in the same way as diabetes: a disease which – if it couldn't be cured – could at least be controlled. At the time Gold was writing, no-one knew what caused cachexia.

Gold investigated, and came to the conclusion that cancer imposes a waste-recycling system on the liver and kidneys. The process works like this: cancer uses glucose as its fuel. The waste product that emerges is lactic acid, which is excreted into the blood system and is taken up by the liver and kidneys. The lactic acid is then converted back into glucose by a process that requires a great deal of energy. The more glucose that is created, the more fuel the cancer has to feed on and the more waste products that return to the liver for reconversion. This process depletes the body and energises the cancer. When the body cannot keep up, the result is cachexia.

Dr Gold looked for a drug that would interfere with this process. He found it – hydrazine sulphate. His experiments showed that hydrazine sulphate did indeed have an effect on the cancer energising process. He also found that it had very few side-effects. That is to say, it was not a very toxic substance in its own right.

His first human guinea pig was a woman who was expected to die within a matter of days from Hodgkin's disease. She was bedridden, and not having eaten much for some time, was 'paper thin'. Administration of the drug resulted in a very quick improvement. Within a week, she was shopping, within five weeks she was pottering about her garden. Dr Dean Burke of the National Cancer Institute in Washington declared: '[Hydrazine sulphate is] the most remarkable anti-cancer agent I have come across in my forty-five years of experience of cancer.'

That was in August 1973. So, why isn't everyone now taking hydrazine sulphate? Because it eventually wound up on the ACS's list of unproven therapies . . . This despite the evidence that Gold put forward to support its value. Gold claimed that out of eighty-four patients with advanced-stage cancer treated by other doctors with hydrazine sulphate, seventy per cent showed subjective improvements (i.e. lessened pain, improved appetite) and seventeen per cent had had objective improvements (tumour regression, disappearance of cancer-related disorders). These are very good figures, given that all the patients were considered terminal and the success rate should therefore have been close to zero.

Russian scientists at the N. N. Petrov Research Institute of Oncology in St Petersburg have replicated these results. In 1974, they used hydrazine sulphate on forty-eight patients considered terminal. They found that almost sixty per cent felt subjectively much better, indeed euphoric! Their appetites improved and the pain lessened or disappeared. Over half of these had clear signs of tumour control. The Russian team also found another interesting attribute of hydrazine sulphate: it appeared to make cancers more vulnerable to chemotherapy, even in the case of tumours that had previously been resistant to chemotherapy.

Support for hydrazine sulphate finally resulted in clinical trials. These have now reached the phase 3 level – the final stage – where human terminally ill cancer patients are studied. Previous studies show that it works against every kind of tumour at every stage. In 1985, Tim Hansen, an eleven-year-old boy with three inoperable brain tumours, was given one week to live. A few weeks later he was put on hydrazine sulphate. He is still taking the hydrazine sulphate as the tumours are still in evidence ten years later – but he is alive.

Gold's recommended dosage for adults weighing over 45 kg (100 lbs) is 60 mg per day for the first three days, then 60 mg twice a day for the next three days, and 60 mg three times a day thereafter. This treatment must continue for as long as there is evidence of a tumour in the body. No dose higher than 60 mg is to be tried, as this can cause nerve damage. Alcohol, tranquillisers and barbiturates must not be taken during the course of the treatment as these inhibit the action of the drug. For patients weighing under 45 kg, the dosage should be halved.

For sources of hydrazine sulphate, see Resources.[35]

Hydrotherapy

Water is a powerful cleaning agent, and the skin is an important organ for the elimination of toxins. Putting these two together, we get hydrotherapy, of which there are many forms. Saunas and steambaths are one. Spending at least half an hour in the heat – but not continuously – for five- to fifteen-minute sessions are the norm. The purpose is not only to sweat out the poisons in the body; the heat also acts as an immune system stimulator.

Some health clinics offer a hydrotherapy treatment involving wrapping the body in hot towels, but a hot bath at home – as hot as can be borne – can work just as well. Add 450 grams (1 lb) of baking soda and 450 grams of sea salt or deep mine salt (not standard table salt, which is totally ineffective). Rock salt is not so good. Stay in the bath for twenty to fifty minutes, and then have a quick shower to rub off the soda and salt. This is known as a detox (detoxification) bath.

It is important with all these forms of hydrotherapy to drink lots of water – distilled or natural spring/mineral water – before, during and after the sessions.

Hypnosis

Hypnosis isn't a 'state' of mind like dream-sleep. It is a condition of mind in which all other mental states can be suggested externally. It is well known that people in a hypnotic trance can turn their hands warm and cold simply by focusing their attention on achieving these changes. Hypnotic suggestion can create even blisters and rashes on the skin.

The mind's brain waves have different frequencies while it is occupying different states. During wakefulness, the brain waves are in the beta range (fourteen cycles per second, or more). In sleep, they are in the alpha range (seven to fourteen cycles per second), occasionally dipping into the delta and theta ranges. Through hypnosis, we are taken into the alpha range while still in a state of wakefulness.

In the alpha state, the subconscious mind is open to suggestive input. Hypnotist William Hewitt refers to the subconscious as 'an obedient slave' that doesn't think or reason: 'It just responds to what it is told. Herein lies the value and power of hypnosis. By hypnosis you can pump powerful suggestions directly into your subconscious. Your subconscious accepts them and causes them to become reality. It is extremely important that all suggestions given are positive, constructive and beneficial.' (William Hewitt, 1994)

In his book, *Hypnosis*, Hewitt discounts some myths. He says that people cannot be hypnotised against their will, because one of the preconditions is complete cooperation. Secondly, the hypnotised person is always aware of what suggestions are being made and any upsetting suggestion would cause the subject to come out of the hypnotic state immediately, of their own choice. According to Hewitt, almost everybody can be hypnotised. In fact, you don't need to go to a hypnotist to be hypnotised – you can hypnotise yourself. However, he suggests that it is easier to do this once you have first been hypnotised by someone else.

There are books about hypnosis and self-hypnosis on the market, certainly in any New Age bookshop you will find books such as the above, or Frank S. Caprio's *Better Health with Self-Hypnosis*.

A CAUTIONARY NOTE
Anyone considering hypnosis should be very aware of the dangers. One girl was seriously injured when told to walk off the edge of a stage by a performing hypnotist. She did so, and broke her back. Another girl was told to imagine she had been hit by a 10,000 volt charge. Shortly afterwards she went home, lay down and died. Anyone visiting a hypnotherapist should specify in advance exactly what messages are to be uttered. It may be advisable to take a companion along to ensure this.

Under hypnosis, people can be made insensible to pain and to carry out tasks that would otherwise be considered impossible. Post-hypnotic suggestions can be implanted, so that a person will carry out a task at some time after emerging from the hypnotic state. Hypnotic states will normally be slept off. In some subjects, hypnosis is so deep that surgery can be performed without anaesthetic. This was first demonstrated in the mid-nineteenth century by a surgeon in Calcutta, James Esdaile.

Iscador
This therapy is closely associated with institutions that follow Rudolf Steiner's anthroposophical movement. It is well

261

known in Germany. Iscador is the trade name for a number of preparations made with different types of mistletoe that grow on different kinds of tree and therefore exhibit different properties. These are further combined with homeopathic doses of such metals as silver, copper and mercury. Although condemned by the American Cancer Society, it is approved for use in Germany and Switzerland. The Lukas Clinic in Arlesheim, Switzerland, is the major centre where this therapy is carried out. However, any doctor can procure the capsules.

Iscador is given by subcutaneous injection at a site close to the tumour, starting with low doses and gradually increasing them until the patient reacts by showing a clear objective or subjective improvement in general health, the tumour slows down or there is a fever reaction.

Does Iscador work? A lot of evidence suggests it does. One of its most obvious effects is that it increases the size of the thymus gland substantially (by nearly one hundred per cent in some animal studies) and the thymus becomes much more active. This is a very significant finding. Iscador works both by attacking the cancer cells directly and by enhancing the immune system. Not all cancers respond well to Iscador – leukaemia, for example. It works best with carcinomas and melanomas.

Although mistletoe is poisonous, Iscador is relatively non-toxic. It is suggested that it can accompany any other anti-cancer treatment as no negative interactions with other medications have been reported. However, it should not be taken by people with heart problems, pregnant women and those taking a prescription drug containing a mono-amineoxidase inhibitor.

It is often combined with a vegetarian diet, excluding mushrooms, tomatoes, new potatoes, sugar, hard fats and alcohol. In addition, patients following an anthroposophical regime are encouraged to engage in artistic activities, including dance, as well as having heat baths, oil baths and massage.

In addition to fighting cancer, Iscador has the effect of aiding sleep, providing pain relief and stimulating weight gain. Many patients report being reinvigorated. See Resources.[36]

The Issels approach
Dr Joseph Issels, working in Bavaria and basing his approach on Max Gerson's work, established what he called

a whole-body therapy to deal with cancer. The therapy is in fact a combination therapy, including ozone-oxygen treatments, diet, fever therapy and even low-dose chemotherapy and radiation.

For Issels, the body has four interrelated defence systems. Firstly, there are the lymphocytes and antibodies normally considered to be the entire immune system. Secondly, there are the eliminating and detoxifying organs: liver, kidneys, skin and intestine. Thirdly, there are the friendly bacteria in the epithelial tissues of the body. Lastly, there is the connective tissue, where organic salts are stored and toxins are digested or bound chemically to make them inert. Issels also made a point of insisting that infected teeth and tonsils should be removed – including all teeth filled with mercury amalgam and teeth whose pulp has been removed through root canal treatment. He believes that these impair the immune system.

External observers have calculated that seventeen per cent of Issels' patients go on to long-term remission. Since most of them were diagnosed as terminal when they arrived at his clinic, this is an excellent result.

Issels was not left free to pursue his own therapies, however, and was blacklisted by the American Cancer Society in 1958. In 1960, he was arrested on charges of fraud, and imprisoned without bail. After five years of court cases, he was finally acquitted of all charges. But in the meantime, his clinic had been forced to close. Although he reopened it, after years of attempts to discredit him by the medical establishment, Issels carried on his work in a much smaller way, finally retiring. Penny Brohn established the Bristol Cancer Help Centre to carry on Issels' kind of work. In Germany, Issels' work is being continued by Dr Wolfgang Woeppel.[37]

Laetrile
Laetrile is the litmus test of all litmus tests. If you find a book on cancer and you wish to know where on the medical spectrum the writer is sitting, the quickest and easiest way is to look up laetrile in the index and read what he or she has to say. If the writer is against it, then the writer is writing from an orthodox position. Those who are for it are generally coming from an alternative viewpoint.

Laetrile is one name given to a substance found in concentrated form in apricot kernels and almonds. Also known as amygdalin, it is found in varying quantities in up to 2,500 other plants, the vast majority of which are edible. In the early seventies, Dr Harold Manner of the Biology Department at Loyola University, Chicago, conducted a study on a strain of mice genetically engineered to produce females that develop spontaneous mammary tumours. Using a combination of enzymes, Vitamin A and laetrile, he reported in his book, *The Death of Cancer*: 'After six to eight days an ulceration appeared at the tumour site. Within the ulceration was a pus-like fluid. An examination of this fluid revealed dead malignant cells. The tumour gradually underwent complete regression in seventy-five of the experimental animals. This represented 89.3 per cent of the total group.' (Quoted in Moss, 1982)

Further tests on 550 mice, comparing enzymes, vitamin A and laetrile alone and in combinations of two, and of all three together, showed that the enzymes alone or in combination with either laetrile or vitamin A produced regression in fifty-two to fifty-four per cent of the mice. Laetrile on its own had no visible effect, but when all three were in combination, there was total regression in thirty-six out of fifty cases – i.e. seventy-two per cent.

Pure laetrile, however, has very recently been taken off the shelves in Britain, having been illegal in much of the US for decades. Opponents of laetrile argue that it is potentially toxic and can lead to cyanide poisoning. However, this can only happen if pure laetrile is taken orally – because any cyanide that is released does so as a result of the action of the digestive enzymes. In the late 1970s, an estimated 50,000–100,000 cancer patients were taking over 1 million grams a month. Only two, or possibly three, deaths from an accidental overdose of this substance have been reported.

Laetrile-rich foods, though, can be eaten more or less with impunity. Almonds and apricots – particularly apricot kernel oil – are eaten in large quantities in the Hunza valley in northern Pakistan. Until modern diets started to impact on the way of life there, cancer was unknown.

Anecdotal evidence from a number of doctors supports the use of laetrile therapy. Leon Chaitow, in his book *An End to Cancer?*, quotes Dutch doctor H. Moolenburgh: 'I have been treating cancer patients for twenty-five years and introduced laetrile four years ago [i.e. in 1973]. That was a turning point. For the first time, I saw people who stayed alive in the late stages of cancer, against all expectations.' In addition: 'A lot of patients with hopeless cancer feel better, have less pain and live longer than I would have expected. And some cases live on and on and on, which could not be expected at all. I did not see that sort of patient before laetrile.'

HOW DOES LAETRILE WORK?
One good description of this process is that laetrile is a parcel that contains poisons. When the parcel is unwrapped, the poisons are released. Normal cells do not have the power to unwrap the parcel. Only cancer cells have that power. Laetrile is a substance that can be separated (by enzymes, in the presence of water) into glucose, benzaldehyde and hydrocyanic acid. The last two substances are each, individually, a poison, but together they work synergistically, i.e. they are more powerful together, in combination, than they are separately. The enzyme that unwraps this package is beta-glucoronidase. This enzyme appears in great quantities in and around cancer cells – but not normal cells. The German doctor, Hans Nieper, argues that a synthetic version of laetrile, mandelonitrile, might be even more effective.

Laetrile apparently works best on slow-growing cancers in the early stages of malignancy. Late stage malignancies need to be slowed down. One way of achieving this is through copper replacement therapy – copper is a vital mineral that is eliminated by cancer cells. Copper supplements help to slow down the respiration rate of the cancer cell, which improves the chances of laetrile working.

Proponents of laetrile therapy insist that tumour regression is only one possible outcome. Pain relief and improved subjective feelings of well-being also result. This well-being is the result of the benzaldehyde, a known pain-killer.

The question of tumour regression is sometimes brought up as evidence that laetrile is ineffective. Laetrile, it appears, does not make tumours grow smaller. At first sight, it seems to make sense that if laetrile does not cause tumours to grow smaller, then this is a clear sign that it is an ineffective anti-cancer agent. This raises an important question about the nature of cancer and tumours.

Laetrilists argue that tumour size is not a good indicator of anti-cancer activity. Their reasoning is as follows. A tumour does not just consist of malignant cells. It also contains a large proportion of normal cells. Chemotherapy attacks all cells, so it is not unusual to see significant short-term tumour regression with chemotherapeutic drugs: they kill the malignant and the normal cells together. However, the long-term result may be, in fact, to make the tumour even more aggressive by increasing the proportion of malignant cells. Laetrile, on the other hand, does not affect the normal cells – only the malignant ones. Therefore the tumour will not decrease in size. It will simply have been made unmalignant. The body of the cancer may remain, but without the engine. This view is supported by research. According to pathologist Gerald Dermer: 'There is a marked discrepancy between ostensible tumor response and actual patient survival. In only about thirty-two per cent of the clinical trials that reported significant tumor responses to new drugs was survival also prolonged.'

Laetrilists are almost universal in saying that laetrile therapy must be accompanied by dietary measures – a raw vegetable diet is generally recommended. In fact, such a diet will contain a large amount of dietary laetrile. Indeed, one of the things that makes the laetrile controversy so bizarre is that laetrile is a very common component of food. Between 1,200 and 2,500 plants contain laetrile – most cereals and fruits and many vegetables. Such ubiquity must have a purpose. However, laetrile remains isolated in an intellectual no-go area by the medical establishment.

A diet that contains good quantities of the following would be high in laetrile: chickpeas, beansprouts, nuts, mung beans, blackberries, raspberries and the seeds of apples, apricots, cherries, plums and pears. Laetrile can be injected or taken orally. Treatment generally consists of 1–2 grams taken orally every day with meals (not more than one gram at any time). Some doctors supplement this with intravenous injections, ranging from 3 grams a week to 9 grams a day (for a short period of a few weeks only). Laetrile is also known as vitamin B17 by those who advocate its use. Note that it deteriorates very fast and so only fresh laetrile should be used.

Those who still need to be convinced of laetrile's safety can take heart from an experiment with mice undertaken at the Sloan-Kettering Center, a leading US cancer research establishment. For thirty months, mice were injected daily with 2 grams per kilogram of laetrile (equivalent to giving a human being 100 grams a day). At the end of the period, these mice were healthier and exhibited better well-being than the control group who did not get any laetrile. How this experiment and other laetrile supporting research got suppressed takes up a fascinating chapter in Ralph Moss's book, *The Cancer Syndrome*.

See Resources for sources of laetrile.[38]

Lakhovsky's cosmic energy cure

Georges Lakhovsky, a Russian engineer living in France, conducted a number of experiments that led him to the belief that all life radiates vibrations, which emanate from the oscillation of minute cellular magnetic fields. Every cell is essentially an electrical circuit with its own electromagnetic field. Ill-health occurs, then, when there is a dis-equilibrium caused by a war of radiations between the natural healthy cells and the radiations emanating from viruses or other invading pathogens. If the invading microbial radiation is stronger, the cells' healthy radiations are affected and are unable to maintain their own proper level of radiation. On the other hand, if the cells' healthy radiations are stronger, the microbe is killed.

From this, it follows that if the body can be flooded with oscillations of the same frequency as that of a healthy cell, then the cells should be able to return to their healthy frequencies and so fight off the disease. For this purpose, Lakhovsky developed an oscillator that emitted radiations of the right frequency and did indeed have the effect of curing geraniums that had developed cancer tumours. However, he did not stop there. Thinking about the source of the energy needed to charge the cells in the first place, he came to the conclusion that it was the energy that streams through the cosmos. It should therefore be possible, he thought, to focus this energy without the help of any artificial machinery.

Lakhovsky made a copper circlet, 30 cm (12 inches) in diameter, and attached it to a support made of ebonite, a material made of black vulcanised rubber, which he stuck into the flower pot. He then took two groups of geraniums. Half he injected with a bacterium that causes cancer – the other half were his controls. When the cancerous growths had developed, he placed the coil round one cancerous plant. After several weeks, he found that all the cancer-infected plants had died – with one exception. The plant in the coil was not only cancer-free, but it had grown twice as large as the normal plants. It was Lakhovsky's view that each healthy vibrating cell responds with its own healthy vibration from the cosmic energy band that contains energy of all possible vibrations.

Subsequently, a number of experiments have been done both with copper circlets in the form of collars, bracelets and belts and with electrical equipment that he designed. These appear to have a profound normalising effect – so making them beneficial for a wide range of illnesses. Even cancer patients experienced speedy remissions. Unfortunately, details of the machine have been largely lost – though some attempts at reconstruction have been made. However, the use of copper circlets is easily achieved. Any length of copper wire can be used – apparently even standard insulated cable. Place circlets round the neck, waist, arms above the elbow and legs above the knee. Secure them in place in any way you can. Since the effect is to normalise the body's natural healthy state by eliminating poisons, some early discomfort may be experienced. A lot of water should be drunk to help the elimination process. Doctors have used these copper circlets in many countries for numerous problems, and no long-term toxic effects have been noted. Short-term effects range from occasional pains and headaches to flu-like symptoms.

See *The Lakhovsky Handbook* and *The Secret of Life* for further details.

Laughter

Laughter is one means by which the body's entire chemistry can be shifted from a state of ill-health to one of health. This was the view of Norman Cousins, who in 1964 found himself in hospital with a profoundly crippling disease which involved the disintegration of the connective tissue of the body. The doctors weren't sure what it was or what to

268

do about it – all they knew was that it was very serious. They could measure how serious it was by testing the sedimentation rate of the red blood cells. The speed with which these cells settle at the bottom of a test-tube measured in millimetres per hour is a sign of health or ill-health. A minor illness will have a sedimentation rate of thirty to forty. Over sixty is serious. Norman Cousins had a sedimentation rate of over eighty.

Cousins quickly decided that hospital was not the right place for him: 'A hospital is no place for a person who is seriously ill. The surprising lack of respect for basic sanitation, the rapidity with which staphylococci and other pathogenic organisms can run around an entire hospital, the extensive and sometimes promiscuous use of X-ray equipment.'

Cousins decided that the reason he had fallen ill was that his adrenal glands had become exhausted. It is known that stress and emotional tension – frustration, rage, etc. – can reduce the functioning of the adrenal glands and the endocrine system to the point where they cannot effectively deal with the toxins in the body caused by these same negative emotions. For Cousins: 'The inevitable question arose in my mind: what about the positive emotions? If negative emotions produce negative chemical changes in the body, wouldn't the positive emotions produce positive chemical changes? Is it possible that love, hope, faith, laughter, confidence, and the will to live have therapeutic value?'

So, Cousins took the brave step of refusing any more pain-killing injections, discharged himself from hospital into a hotel and arranged for a movie projector to be installed. He then set about watching every comic film and television programme he could lay his hands on. When he wasn't watching films, he was reading cartoons. Although his pain was initially all but crippling, he found that laughter gave him real relief. Ten minutes of laughter allowed him two hours of pain-free sleep. It also led to a drop of five points on the sedimentation scale – and this improvement was cumulative.

Cousins supplemented the programme of laughter with large doses of vitamin C, which he took by intravenous drip. He started at 10 grams and built up to 25 grams. Again, it had a measurable effect on the sedimentation rate.

Norman Cousins went on to recover, although the after-effects of his illness stayed with him for years. He wrote up the full story in his book, *An Anatomy of an Illness as Perceived by the Patient.*

Although Cousins did not have cancer, the factors that led to his illness are the very same ones that are implicated in cancer: stress, anxiety and so on, leading to a state of adrenal exhaustion. Also, the blood sedimentation rate is a measure of general health – and general health in Cousins' case led to specific improvements relating to a specific disease. If it can work with one disease, it can work with all diseases.

Live cell therapy

This therapy involves the injection of foetal or embryonic cells from various animals into the body. It is proposed that this can help regenerate tissue. It is claimed that injected liver cells will go to help the liver and that injected kidney cells will go to the patient's kidneys. Using radioactive tracers, this effect was demonstrated at Heidelberg University by Professor Lettré. A key target for this therapy is the thymus gland, so patients receive intramuscular injections of calf thymus glands. There is experimental evidence that some diseases do respond to this treatment. In 1981, the *New England Journal of Medicine* reported that ten out of seventeen children with histiocytosis-X, an immune suppressing disease, recovered after daily injections of thymus extract from five-day-old calves.

It is considered to be helpful for cancer patients – especially for those with early stage cancers who have not had chemotherapy or radiation – but not so effective for terminal cases. This treatment is given at the American Biologics clinic in Tijuana (see Mexican clinics below). Fresh cells must be used, as freeze-dried or nitrogen-frozen cells are believed to lose their effectiveness. Shark embryo cells are also used.

A WARNING

Anyone undergoing such treatments should be aware that German studies have linked the therapy to a large number of fatal or otherwise serious allergic and other reactions. These deaths are blamed on over-use of the therapy.

However, Dr Kuhnau at American Biologics says that his cancer patients receive only three injections, once a week, then two others at three months and six months. Dr Kuhnau has treated over 20,000 patients with this therapy over forty years, and reports no toxic effects greater than some fatigue. This therapy is under attack from animal rights activists and from scientists who fear that infection can indeed be spread in this way from animals to humans.

The Livingston approach

Dr Virginia Livingston, like Roy Rife and Gaston Naessens (see below), took as her starting point the belief that a microbe – one that could change shape – was the cause of cancer. She saw this microbe in 1947, and from then on directed all her work to combating it. She named the microbe 'progenitor cryptocides' (meaning 'hidden, ancestral killer'). Livingston believed that everyone had this microbe, but that it was held in check by the immune system until the system was weakened by stress, diet, or even surgery or other traumatic events. Then it multiplies in overwhelming numbers, becoming invasive and promoting the growth of cancer tumours.

Livingston and her researchers have demonstrated that solutions containing progenitor cryptocides but free of bacteria, sealed off from external contamination, subsequently become populated by bacteria, proving that the microbe changes form. Such organisms have also been associated with arthritis and multiple sclerosis. She discovered that the microbe secreted a growth hormone identical to that which coats the placenta surrounding a foetus. She believes that this hormone, human chorionic gonadotrophin (HCG), also coats tumour cells. The purpose of the hormone is to alert the immune system not to interfere with the contents of the HCG-coated bundle. Clearly, some biochemical signal is needed to prevent the body's immune system from attacking a new foetus. This, according to Livingston, is it. This has since been confirmed by other researchers.

HCG has to be kept in check by antibodies, or it will grow out of control. One substance that neutralises it is abscisic acid. Foods rich in abscisic acid are: carrots, mangoes, avocados, tomatoes, lima beans and green leaf vegetables. Since the liver's ability to break down vitamin A is impaired,

271

Livingston mixes dried liver powder with it, and this does the liver's job. In the body, abscisic acid's purpose is to break down vitamin A into a number of retinoids which are growth inhibitors and which regulate HCG. For this reason, too much carrot juice or vitamin A could be dangerous for pregnant women and those considering pregnancy.

Livingston's regime is to rebuild the immune system with a vegetarian raw food diet, vitamin and mineral supplements, gamma globulin injections and – the key differentiating element of the therapy – an autogenous vaccine given in conjunction with a BCG vaccination. The therapy forbids chicken, beef, eggs and milk. One animal husbandry expert, Elizabeth McCulloch, believes that as many as forty per cent of human cancers are caused by active cancer-causing microbes transmitted directly from eggs and chickens. Other experts, while avoiding pointing the finger of blame at chickens, agree that at least thirty per cent of cancers are caused by viruses. In Sweden and Switzerland, milk from leukaemia-infected cattle is not allowed to reach the market. This is not the case in the UK or the US.

How effective is the therapy? Livingston claimed an eighty per cent remission rate. Other studies suggest that her treatment is no improvement on orthodox treatment – but that does not mean it is any less effective.

In 1968, without conducting any form of test, and without any evidence from any other research, the ACS put the Livingston vaccine on its list of unproven therapies. In February 1990, Dr Livingston was ordered to stop using this vaccine, as it had not been shown to be safe and effective. There had been no complaints from patients.

See Resources for the Livingston Foundation Medical Center.[39]

Maharishi Ayurvedic therapy

Maharishi Mahesh Yogi gained instant fame from his association with the Beatles and other pop icons of the 1960s. He launched the Transcendental Meditation Movement, and then established a number of Maharishi Ayurvedic health centres, most of which are in America.

Anyone seeking help from these centres will be put on a gentle regime involving a change of diet, Ayurvedic herbs, a daily routine of exercises, and instruction in Transcendental

Meditation. As Dr Deepak Chopra, who used to work at the Maharishi Ayurveda Health Center in Lancaster, Massachusetts, says: 'In Ayurveda, a level of total, deep relaxation is the most important precondition for curing any disorder. The body knows how to maintain balance unless thrown off by disease; therefore, if one wants to restore the body's own healing ability, everything should be done to bring it back into balance.'

The Ayurvedic approach to healing also includes two other techniques which Chopra reports, but does not describe. One is primordial sound therapy and the other is the bliss technique. Primordial sound therapy assumes that underlying all matter there are vibrations of energy which can be heard when the meditating person is still and the mind is quiet: 'The theory behind primordial sound treatment is that the mind can return to the quantum level, introduce certain sounds that may have become distorted along the way, and thus have a profound healing influence in the body.'

The bliss technique is a method for allowing the flow of joyful energy by the use of what Chopra calls a 'faint mental impulse', which helps the mind come into contact with 'the vibrations of bliss that subtly pervade every cell of the body. In and of itself, this feeling is extremely pleasant, but it also indicates that quantum healing is taking place, that disrupted channels of inner intelligence are being repaired. When these channels are closed, bliss cannot flow. When they are open, contact with the quantum mechanical body is restored.'

To learn more of these techniques, you should write to any of the centres listed in Chopra's book, *Perfect Health*, or see Resources.[40]

Massage

The human touch has great power to heal – and the lack of touch has great power to kill. A century ago, it was a well-known but little understood fact that young infants in institutions and orphanages had a high death rate. Doctors called it marasmus. These institutions were run, like many such places even today, in an efficient, no-nonsense way. In the 1930s, a new view of how young children should be brought up came to the fore. 'Mothering' became accepted – children were hugged, fondled and bounced up and down. The result was that the death rate fell to a fraction of what it had been.

Massage is known to help reduce pain. It increases relaxation and, at the same time, increases energy levels, ridding the body of tiredness.

Physiotherapists today are lineal descendants of massagers of the last century, but as this discipline has become more mechanistic and scientific, it has tended to leave the massaging skills behind. Massage, sadly, has acquired an unsavoury reputation because of its euphemistic use in the sex industry. But it has a very important place in the health practices of the Turks, Arabs, Indians and Chinese. The simple fact is, a massage makes you feel good, and that sense of feeling good is fundamental to good health.

For people with cancers, there may be good reasons for not having a massage. One obvious reason is that a hard massage may inadvertently help the cancer cells to spread through the lymphatic system. However, this caution does not apply to aromatherapy and relaxation massages, which tend to be softer.

Meditation

Most people think of meditating as a way of relaxing and emptying the mind. Such meditation masters as Maharishi Yogi laugh at this way of describing it, however. For them, it is a way of entering a state of consciousness where other energy fields can be experienced. And these can only be experienced in the silence of the mind. It is now known that meditation is a state of consciousness that is different from being awake, from being asleep and from dreaming. This fourth state is a measurable one. Machines designed to measure brain waves can distinguish the state of meditation from the other three states.

The tradition of meditation originated in India, where it is known as *dhyan*, a term meaning to bring the mind to rest in the silence of the fourth state. Dr Deepak Chopra describes it like this: 'The whole phenomenon is an immediate experience, like recognising the fragrance of lilacs or the sound of a friend's voice. It is immediate, non-verbal, and, unlike a flower's fragrance, totally transforming.'

In meditation, the meditator feels a heightened sense of awareness and inner silence. Robert Keith Wallace, at

UCLA, found that people who meditate regularly become physiologically younger than those who don't. For the first five years, each year of meditation has the effect of making the meditator grow approximately one year younger. After that the rejuvenating process appears to speed up.

A 1986 study by the Blue Cross Shield insurance company found that people who meditate have less than half the number of tumours among non-meditators. A 1979 Israeli study found that meditation helps people with abnormally high cholesterol levels to lower these levels and so reduce their risk of heart attack.

How can you learn to meditate? There are a number of different forms of meditation, of which the best-known is Transcendental Meditation (TM). People involved in TM insist that it must be learned from an authorised instructor as there are subtleties that need to be explored. However, many people find that they can meditate perfectly well by following a few basic steps. The general principles of all meditation are to sit quietly in a chair with eyes closed. A special word or mantra – words selected for their sound – is repeated by the mind, and the mind is led by the sound to the inner silences of the mind. In TM, the instructor will provide a mantra, but some studies on meditation have found that almost any word will do: e.g. peace, let go, relax or just mmm. The most famous mantra of all is Om Mani Padme Hum – or simply Om for short.

One guide to good meditation practice recommends these steps:

1. Choose a quiet spot where you will not be disturbed.
2. Sit in a comfortable position with a straight back. Some people like to cross their ankles.
3. Close your eyes.
4. Relax your muscles from head to feet by focusing the mind on the tip of the nose. Then let the mind travel up the nose, round the face and skull to the back of the neck, then slowly round the shoulders and arms, the back, the buttocks, the legs and the feet. Become aware of any tensions, and with the help of the mind, induce relaxation in these places.
5. Become aware of the breathing, watching it go in and out, without any desire to control it.

6. Repeat the word you have chosen as your focus word or mantra.
7. If you become aware that your thoughts have drifted, stop the thoughts and return to your mantra.
8. Practise every day for fifteen to twenty minutes.
9. Do not judge anything about the performance. In meditation, things just happen. It is important to be aware of this, and to accept that they are happening – even to understand what is happening – but do not be in any way critical or judgmental.

Melatonin

Until recently, the functions of the pineal gland have remained pretty much a mystery. However, melatonin, the pineal gland's chief hormone, is now receiving a lot of attention. For one thing, it is now known to regulate the circadian rhythm, the body's biological clock. It is used as an antidote to jet-lag and as a supplement that is helpful in reducing anxiety, panic attacks and migraines, in addition to being an effective sleeping pill, especially as a safe way to get insomniac children to sleep. It does not have the side-effects of other sleeping pills and does not interfere with REM (rapid eye movement) dream states.

However, new studies are suggesting that it has a more powerful part to play in promoting physical health. It has been suggested that melatonin also bolsters the immune system, keeps our cells in a good state of repair, slows the growth of tumours and cataracts and keeps heart disease at arm's length. As one cellular biologist who takes 1 mg every night said in a *Newsweek* article in August 1995: 'I want to die young as late in life as possible, and I think this hormone could help.'

Studies of rats reveal melatonin to be a very potent protector against toxins and radiation that kill by causing DNA damage. It has also helped mice survive infection with the encephalitis virus. Women who want a relatively safe contraceptive could explore the idea of taking high levels of melatonin (75–100 mg per day). An Italian study has shown that a nightly 10 mg dose has significantly improved one-year survival rates of metastatic lung cancer.

To be effective, melatonin must be taken at night, before going to bed. Most people get good effects from doses of

1–10 mg, but there is no sign of any toxicity at higher doses. No scientist has yet developed a concentration capable of killing a mouse; human volunteers who took 6 grams a day for a month merely reported some stomach discomfort and residual sleepiness.

Unfortunately, at the time of writing, melatonin is only freely available in the US, and can be purchased from American sources. Note that this is one of the only supplements that might benefit from being taken in time-release form.

Mexican clinics

Because the medical climate in the US is so hostile to all forms of alternative medicine, Americans seeking access to such treatments have had to cross the border into Mexico. The town of Tijuana is now home to a fair number of clinics specialising in many different approaches, from Hoxsey's Herbs and the Gerson diet to magnets and Rife generators. For addresses of some of these clinics see Resources.[41]

Oxygen therapy

We have already discussed the relevance of oxygen to cancer. Cancers often, if not always, are generated by tissue conditions of low-oxygenation. In addition, they tend to thrive in these conditions. Consequently, it has been proposed that cancer tumours can be effectively prevented and treated by increasing the oxygen levels of the blood and tissues.

The problem is exacerbated by the decreasing oxygen levels in the air. Studies of air trapped in Arctic ice show that the oxygen levels of the air have decreased from over thirty per cent a century ago to under twenty per cent nowadays. Fluoridated water slows down the body's uptake of oxygen. Poor food, poor eating practices – fast eating, overeating – lack of exercise, bad breathing techniques, all worsen the problem. It is argued that good mental attitudes and meditation work partly because they lead to more relaxed and deeper breathing. The result is that the oxygen level in ill people is very much lower than that of well people.

A number of ways of achieving higher oxygen levels in the

body have been used – apparently with the sort of success that validates the theory.

Haematogenic Oxidation Therapy (HOT) is one variation. It is a simple and painless method of treatment. A quantity of blood, 100–200 millilitres (about 3½–7 fl oz), is taken from the patient, and oxygen is then bubbled through it. The blood is then irradiated with ultra-violet rays for five to ten minutes, and left to settle for an hour before being returned to the patient by drip. This is a form of ozone therapy. According to Issels, who used this therapy:

> [The blood] is: sterilized, normalized, regenerated and reactivated. Defense cells regain their aggressive capacity. Returned to the host, these cells can once more attack microbes and cancer-promoting viruses which are characterized by an anaerobic metabolism – making them unable to survive in the actively oxidized environment that HOT creates.

This treatment is generally done on a weekly basis, for two to three months, or as long as it takes to achieve the desired result.

Ozone is a very powerful sterilising and cleansing agent. The tap water in most continental European towns and cities is ozonated rather than chlorinated, as are most German public swimming pools. Ozone is a strong anti-carcinogen, while chlorine can – under certain circumstances – promote cancer. Ozone is a far more powerful agent than oxygen, probably because it is highly unstable and releases a lot of energy as it transforms into ordinary oxygen molecules. In 1980, *Science* reported a study into the effects of ozonated air on cancer cells. The growth of the cancer cells was inhibited by ninety per cent. Ozone has also been implicated in dramatic success stories in the fight against AIDS.

Ozone therapy is very common in Germany, and at Dr Renate Viebahn's clinic in Iffezheim, patients are given intramuscular ozone injections. German practitioners now recommend that ozone should be given in doses not higher than 100 micrograms per millilitre, as more can be damaging to normal cells. Ozone treatments also start with small doses and build up in strength slowly. How dangerous is it? According to author Ed McCabe in Germany, 644 therapists

278

reported using ozone therapy on 384,775 patients. They received a total of 5.5 million ozone treatments, and the incidence of negative side-effects was 0.0007 per cent.

A form of increasingly common treatment is to have humidified ozone applied either vaginally, or through the rectum, in short thirty-second to one-minute bursts. This allows a very rich ozone concentration to be absorbed by the blood in a painless, non-invasive way.

HYDROGEN PEROXIDE

Another form of hyper-oxygenation therapy is through the use of hydrogen peroxide, intravenous H_2O_2. This was first used during the 1918 influenza outbreak. It then became widely used for a variety of viral and bacterial illnesses, with good results. In fact it was the preferred form of treatment until antibiotics arrived on the scene. The body itself manufactures hydrogen peroxide as a first line of defence against toxins and other invaders.

Hydrogen peroxide can be taken in many ways. Doctors prefer to give it in the form of an intravenous drip, which is probably the best method when chronic illness is being treated. However, it can be taken at home in other ways.

It is important to note that hydrogen peroxide, in strengths greater than three per cent, is dangerous. It can normally be bought in strengths of three or six per cent from any chemist shop. Food grade hydrogen peroxide is thirty-five per cent. This is the purest form, and many advocates of hydrogen peroxide therapy urge users to use food grade H_2O_2 for internal use. But it must be diluted! Undiluted H_2O_2 is extremely dangerous.

Hydrogen peroxide can be taken orally, added to a bath, rubbed on the skin or gargled as a mouth wash. One person using regular H_2O_2 is Dr Christiaan Barnard, who takes it for his arthritis. In a letter dated 10 March 1986, he wrote: 'It is true I have found relief from the arthritis and I attribute this to taking hydrogen peroxide orally several times each day.' Suggested quantities are as follows:

FOR ORAL USE (EITHER FOR DRINKING OR MOUTHWASH)

Thirty-five per cent food grade; increasing daily from 1 drop to 25 drops in a glass of water. However, it appears that not many people can tolerate 25 drops in a glass of water. Six per cent solution: $\frac{1}{2}$ teaspoon to 2 teaspoons in a 200 ml (7 floz) glass of water. Three per cent solution: should be mixed one part to five parts of water and then drunk slowly, increasing from 25 to 125 grams (1–4 oz) a day. This regime can be increased to 125 grams three times a day, for a week at a time. This depends on whether it is being taken for curative or maintenance reasons. A maintenance programme of 125 grams a day, two days a week is recommended.

Not everyone agrees that hydrogen peroxide should be taken orally. There are arguments about its effects on stomach acidity and bacteria. There is also the question of whether it can be properly absorbed into the bloodstream in this way, or whether it is broken down to oxygen and water in the stomach. There is general agreement that hydrogen peroxide should not be persisted with if it is uncomfortable. Dr Donsbach, of the Hospital Santa Monica, argues that a preferable way of getting the peroxide effect without the discomfort is to take the same quantity of magnesium peroxide (magnesium dioxide) instead.

H_2O_2 should be taken on an empty stomach, and at least an hour should separate its use and intake of vitamin C, as they negate each other.

FOR USE IN BATHS
Half a cup of food grade thirty-five per cent, or 600 ml (1 pint) of three per cent can be added to half a bath of water. Soak for twenty minutes, and it is claimed you will feel rejuvenated. To give an indication of how powerful the skin is as an absorbing organ, a 90 kg (200 lb) person can absorb up to 1.8 kg (4 lb) of water from a twenty-minute soak in a bath.

CONTRAINDICATIONS AND A CAUTION
Hydrogen peroxide should not be taken by anyone who has had a transplanted organ. Rejection of the organ may result. A drop of food grade H_2O_2 on the skin will cause a white burn mark. Anyone with children should not have it around the house.[42]

Photodynamic therapy
Can cancer be killed by a death ray? In his book, *Light: Medicine of the Future*, Jacob Liberman reported that over

3,000 people with a variety of malignant tumours had been treated with a method known as photodynamic therapy, and that the results had been very exciting: 'Although they had been treated previously with surgery, chemotherapy, radiation, immunotherapy or a combination of these, their tumours responded positively to the light treatment seventy or eighty per cent of the time, *after only one treatment.*' (Author's italics)

This therapy is based on two facts. The first is that there is a family of substances known as porphyrins which, when injected into the body, are selectively taken up by cancer cells – but not by most normal cells. The interesting thing about porphyrins is that they are light-sensitive to a high degree. They are not toxic in the dark, but are highly toxic in the light. The second fact is that when the cancer cells have taken up the porphyrins, they will fluoresce under ultraviolet light. This allows their position to be ascertained with a high degree of accuracy, if they are not too deeply embedded in tissue.

Using this information, cancer patients are injected with porphyrins and then, once the sites of the cancer cells have been located, a red light – tuned to a wavelength of 630 nanometres – is delivered, using an argon pumped laser, directly to the treatment site; the fibreoptic tube used is no thicker than a hair. 'Within hours of the light treatment, the cancer cells begin to die, leaving most normal tissues unharmed. Even in tissues that are just partially cancerous, only the cancerous portion of the tissue will die. Since specific photosensitive dyes are combined with highly tuned laser light, the treatment is extremely precise.' (Liberman, 1991)

One problem with this therapy is that the liver, kidneys and spleen also retain porphyrins. For this reason, a gap of twenty-four to seventy-two hours between injecting the porphyrins and turning on the red light is left, to allow the normal tissues to clear out the porphyrins. In addition, patients undergoing this treatment suffer from increased skin sensitivity to sunlight, which may result in intense skin irritation for four to six weeks after treatment.

Apart from these two problems, this therapy appears to offer an extremely good method of ridding the body of the tumour. It remains to be seen whether it will be given the green light of approval by the governing medical bodies in the US.

Posture therapies

It is accepted that there is a close correlation between physical and mental trauma and cancer. This suggests that physical and mental trauma should be dealt with as a potential threat of major proportions to the health.

If we accept that mind and body are one, then it makes sense to see the body as a memory system for the mind. Negative thoughts affect the way the muscles are used; the more they are used in a particular way, certain postures result that can lead to postural imbalances, which in themselves will have other negative effects on health. Physical traumas too are, it seems, retained in the body long after the original 'insult' (to use the medical term) appears to have been healed.

Another argument in favour of having good posture is that it will benefit breathing, which in turn will influence the amount of oxygen in our blood and tissues.

Kinesiology is one of a number of postural retraining therapies. It involves training the patient in the proper use of the body in posture movement and repose, in order to achieve healing. The principle behind it is that mental as well as physical energy is tied up in inappropriate postures and actions. Poor posture and lack of proper exercise puts a strain on the body. However, by using the body properly, we can relieve this stress. Swinging and swaying can loosen up the joints. Jarring and jolting movements need to be avoided. To straighten the spine using simple traction, you can hang your head over the end of your bed. Movements should, where possible, be slow and harmonious.

The Alexander Technique was developed by an Australian, Frederick Alexander. According to Alexander, 'use affects function'. Ill-use distorts and misshapes the body and interferes with free functioning. When Professor Tinbergen gave his Nobel Prize speech in 1973 (he won the prize for medicine), he used this forum to praise Alexander's work.

American Ida Rolf developed a system known today as rolfing. It is more concerned with structure and bodily mechanics than with posture and movement.

Osteopathy was developed by Dr Andrew Taylor Still (1828–1917), a physician from Missouri who developed a system of treatment without drugs. He believed that ill health was the result of blockages to the circulatory and nervous systems. All the doctor has to do is to make sure these are cleared, and mother nature will do the rest. Surprisingly to the modern reader, he was very effective in curing infectious diseases.

Many modern osteopaths have retreated from this system, so the fact that a practitioner is a Doctor of Osteopathy is no guarantee that he or she uses a drugless medicine based on manipulation. Anyone seeking an osteopath should first ascertain whether or not they use cranial therapy. Cranial therapists believe that through cranial manipulation they can release blockages that impede the flow of living energy that is the essential feature of health and life. Dr Andrew Weil, in his book *Spontaneous Healing*, described his observations of an osteopath working in this way. Originally sceptical, he came away from the experience with the belief that everyone the man had 'fixed' had indeed been made well.

Chiropractic is a more muscular and no-nonsense approach to fixing the joints in the spine and neck. Nevertheless, it too can claim its share of success in solving problems arising from physical trauma.

It seems clear that manipulating the body is an effective way of dealing with a wide range of ills and the surprise is that it has not been taken up in any way by orthodox practitioners of medicine.

Potassium

Sodium and potassium tend to compete within the body. If the body's tissues are high in sodium, then the tissues will not take up proper amounts of potassium. The problem is that sodium is 'bad' and potassium is 'good'. It is important to maintain a low-sodium/high-potassium balance in the body. Good amounts of vitamin B6 are also important to help regulate the balance. According to Dr Tresillian Fere, cancer is the result of the body's inability to process the amount of sodium in the body. High sodium levels in the blood cause low potassium levels, with a consequent impact on blood sugar levels, which drop. Potassium is also lost in the urine when a person is under stress.

A healthy diet should therefore be rich in foods that are high in potassium, or a regular potassium supplement needs to be taken. Potassium rich foods are: almonds, apricots, avocados, bananas, lima, mung and pinto beans, dates, dried figs, hazelnuts, raw garlic, raw horseradish, raw parsley, rice bran, soybeans, full fat soybean flour, sunflower seeds, kelp, blackstrap molasses and brewer's yeast. (The latter three are the richest sources of potassium.)

Prayer

In one study, investigators asked people who had undergone remarkable recovery which activities they believed had most helped. Prayer came out on top of the list, at sixty-eight per cent, followed by meditation and exercise (sixty-four per cent), visualisation (fifty-nine per cent), walking (fifty-two per cent), music/singing (fifty per cent) and other forms of stress reduction (fifty per cent).

We can consider prayer's possible benefits in a number of ways. It may be effective psychologically for the praying person to pray for him or herself. By praying, the person can release thoughts and feelings within. Or, if faith is great, there may be a conviction that God will intercede, creating a placebo effect. Most people will accept that prayer can be very beneficial under these circumstances.

What of prayer acting at a distance, the prayer for one person by another? Such ideas are as old as man. One thousand years ago, the great Persian doctor, Avicenna, wrote: 'The imagination of man can act not only on his own body but even other and very distant bodies. It can fascinate and modify them; make them ill, or restore them to health.' Such an idea is now equated with witchcraft, sorcery, shamanism or just plain superstition. But was Avicenna right? Is there any evidence that prayer can work?

There is, in fact, evidence of a kind. Some studies indicate that people directing simple clear messages can often have a measurable physiological effect on other people, plants or objects. What is more, it appears that this gift is a widespread one, and not the preserve of a small group who are psychically skilled.

In one study, ten people tried to inhibit the growth of fungus cultures in the laboratory by consciously focusing their thoughts for fifteen minutes from a distance of approximately one metre. The cultures were then incubated for several more hours. Of a total of 194 culture dishes, 151 showed retarded growth. In a further study, one group of people demonstrated the same effect – inhibiting the growth of the fungus – in sixteen out of sixteen trials, while stationed from one to fifteen miles away from the fungus cultures.

Of course, these two studies show that negative thoughts have the same power as positive thoughts. In another experiment, a healer showed that he could affect the molecular bonding of water molecules by concentrating his mind.

However, according to Dr Larry Dossey, prayers are more likely to be beneficial if they are undirected and are accompanied by complete acceptance of the situation. 'Do with me what you will' is more likely to be effective than 'Dear God, please cure me of my cancer in my left breast.' Certainly, it is a fact that can be subjectively confirmed, that the mind is more deeply and more wholly at peace when it utters the former prayer than when it utters the latter. It seems almost as if a different, deeper, more pleasure-related part of the mind is engaged.

Dossey also thinks that our hidden thoughts and feelings about other people may have the power to harm or heal unconsciously. If this is the case, are patients affected by their doctor's belief systems? If the doctor is thinking: this woman will die in three months' time, will that affect the outcome? Again, many people are convinced that the doctor's negative thoughts may have a negative effect on the prognosis.

We should, however, also consider the fact that if all our individual prayers were answered, the world would be in a sorry state. If every Indian and Chinese father praying for a son was granted his wish, the entire Indian and Chinese people would be dead in a generation.

Psychic surgery

Psychic surgery is practised widely in Brazil and the Philippines. And despite investigations that appear to expose them as frauds, practitioners have a good record of healing. They appear to perform surgery with their bare hands, or with

285

rusty knives, without anaesthesia and without pain. The hand appears to delve into the flesh and a bloody lump of flesh appears in the psychic surgeon's palm. Hocus pocus? Quackery? Some investigators say they are out-and-out frauds, who use magic sleight of hand to pluck out what appear to be cancerous tumours, but which are in fact concealed lumps of chicken or cow flesh. Perhaps. But even so, they have a very potent weapon that the modern scientific doctor denies himself: the psychic surgeons are working with the placebo effect and not against it.

Nevertheless, they remain an enigma. The placebo effect cannot explain all that they do. One famous Brazilian healer worked without touching his patients – he would write down prescriptions as patients filed past. In one test, 1,000 patients filed past. Later, his diagnoses were, according to the report, found to be phenomenally accurate. This ability should not be easily dismissed as impossible. In 1985, an American doctor, Norman Shealy, began to work with a journalist, Caroline Myss, who claimed she had always had an intuitive ability to 'know' things. They lived more than 1,000 miles apart. He would phone her and ask her to help him diagnose the state of health of the patient in his room. Once she was comfortable with this procedure, she would intuitively enter the patient's body, travelling through it to assess the health of each specific organ. According to Shealy, her diagnoses were ninety-three per cent accurate.

Biologist Lyall Watson studied a psychic healer in the Philippines. The man would point his finger about an inch from the patient's skin and an incision would appear. One day, Watson got too close – his own hand was caught in the path, and he got cut.

A final anecdotal note. My otherwise sceptical physiotherapist aunt had a friend with breast cancer, who travelled to the Philippines to visit one of these healers. Her tumour disappeared . . .

Reducing stress

The connection between stress and disease has been recognised for centuries. In 1402, an Italian doctor wrote to his patient: 'Let me speak to you regarding the things you must beware. To get angry and shout at times pleases me, for this will keep up your natural heat; but what displeases me is your being grieved and taking all things to heart. For it is this, as the whole physic teaches, which destroys our body more than any other cause.' This ancient Italian doctor recognised that having a good shout or temper tantrum was stress-relieving, and that dwelling on problems was not healthy.

The connection between stress and cancer has been demonstrated by injecting experimental animals with cortisone, the stress hormone. Animals injected with cortisone have a higher cancer incidence than controls. There is a theory that the seeds of the cancer process are constantly present, but that they are detected and destroyed by the immune system before they can proceed. However, this surveillance system may be adversely affected by prolonged stress caused by fear, anger, depression or other negative emotions over a long period of time.

In one study, it was found that those who viewed their lives as difficult and unsatisfactory and who had a rigid or obsessive attitude towards responsibilities, goals and duties were most often ill, while those who saw their lives as satisfactory and were flexible and open in their approach to responsibilities and duties were least often ill.

Other predictors of stress-related ill-health are constant anxiety or repressed anger. These can be combated through exercise, good breathing habits, a change of diet, supplementation with melatonin and psychotherapeutic activities, such as those mentioned elsewhere in this part of the book. A good technique for speedy relaxation is to pull in the stomach muscles sharply and then to let them out. Repeated a number of times, this gets rid of muscular tension.

Some individuals are apparently more stress-hardy than others. They resist the impact of stress better. Studies into what makes people stress-hardy show that they tend to be people who demonstrate three characteristic attitudes:

1. Commitment, defined as having an attitude of curiosity and involvement in whatever is happening.
2. Control, defined as a belief that we can influence events, coupled with the willingness to act on that belief rather than be a victim of circumstances.
3. A sense of challenge in the face of the obstacles and changes that we all experience.

People who demonstrate these three attitudes demonstrate a healthy desire to engage. People with this mind-set are proofed against illness. Those who demonstrate the opposite attitudes of fearfulness, helplessness and alienation are the most likely to fall ill when stressful events arise.

Reflexology

Foot massages have been known to have a beneficial relaxing effect since time began. The present-day system of reflexology arose as a result first of the work of Dr William Fitzgerald in 1913. He came to the view that there were ten vertical zones running down the body. After further experimentation, he found that by putting pressure on a specific area of the body, he could anaesthetise related areas along the zone. This early work was developed by Eunice Ingham in the 1930s. She found that working on the feet alone was the same as working on the whole body. (Note that acupuncturists also recognise that the foot, hand, ears and other places are microsystems that mirror the workings of the entire body – as a result, some acupuncturists only work on the ear, no matter what or where the ailment is.)

Modern reflexologists have mapped out very precise points on the soles and sides of the feet that correspond to the different organs of the body. If there is a problem in any of the organs, small crystalline deposits can be felt in the related areas in the feet. The massage eliminates these crystal deposits, and this has a healing effect on the organ concerned. As with acupuncture, one way to find areas where there might be a health concern is to test for sensitivity. Any sensitivity is a sign that attention is needed.

Reflexologists do not diagnose specific illnesses, though they will say which tissues or organs are in need of attention. Clearly, while not being specifically an anti-cancer therapy, reflexology can play a useful role as part of a bundle of therapies aimed at improving overall health.

Reiki and therapeutic touch

This is a non-contact therapy in which the reiki healer focuses healing energy from the palms of his or her hands on the area of an illness, or on places on the meridians of the body. As with all Chinese-based healing systems, the body is viewed as being filled with channels, known as meridians, of living energy, qi. It is the healer's job to invigorate the flow of this energy, and to remove blockages in the meridians.

The position of the meridians is very precisely known to Chinese healers, but Western doctors are bemused by them, as there is nothing in their knowledge that conforms to the meridians – they do not follow the circulatory or nervous system, for example. However, recently, French researchers injecting radioactive isotopes into human subjects found that they travelled along the lines of the meridians. Also, researchers in bio-magnetism say that the energy flow along the meridians is the way in which the body's magnetic system completes its cycle. The brain pulses a negative magnetic impulse, which travels down the spine and then returns to the brain, along the meridians, through the flesh and organs of the body, in order to complete the circuit.

Reiki is not the only name given to this form of healing – qigong masters also use it, and in the US there is a technique known as therapeutic touch, which despite its name does not involve physical contact.

One clinical test to assess the effectiveness of therapeutic touch was conducted by New York University researcher, Daniel Wirth, in a double-blind study involving forty-four patients with full-skin-thickness surgical wounds, cut deliberately for the purposes of the study. The subjects inserted the arm with the wound through a hole in a wall. They could not see what was happening on the other side. They were told that their 'bio-potential' – a phrase thought up by the doctors to sound important but vague – was being measured by a non-contact device, a procedure lasting five minutes each time. Half the patients received non-contact therapeutic touch treatment, and half held their arm into an empty room. A doctor who did not know which patients were receiving the treatment was delegated to measure the wounds with a highly accurate digital device. There was no placebo effect involved, because there was no suggestion that any healing was taking place. By day sixteen, more than half of the treated group had completely healed (wound size zero) while none of the untreated group had healed.

In another case demonstrating the healing powers of what is known as 'laying on of hands', a Lutheran nun in Darmstadt, Germany, was helping to build a chapel, when she had a bad fall which resulted in a compound pelvic fracture. The nuns maintained a constant vigil for two days and then, against the doctor's advice, took her out of hospital. They prayed and performed laying on of hands. Immediately after the laying on of hands, the nun stood up and announced that she was free of pain. After two weeks, she presented herself back at the hospital and the doctors had to agree that she was cured. This is one of a number of modern miracles presented in an article appearing in the *British Medical Journal* in 1983, by Dr Rex Gardner of Sunderland General Hospital.

The Rife square-wave frequency generator

Royal Raymond Rife was a San Diego inventor who, in the 1920s and 1930s, built an extraordinarily powerful light microscope with a magnification of 60,000X, which made it possible to study living bacteria and viruses. This was a remarkable development that has, since then, been completely ignored. Scientists like their bacteria dead.

As a result of watching living bacteria, Rife saw something very interesting – the bacteria could change their forms from bacillus, to a fungus, to a virus. In all, he identified four forms, one of which – the monococcoid – he found in ninety per cent of cancer patients. Another – the BX form – was, he claimed, the form in which it caused cancer. Any of the forms could change into a BX form within thirty-six hours.

The idea that relatively harmless bacteria can change into cancer-causing viruses is utterly rejected by most scientists – but Rife is not alone in his belief. He is supported by Dr Virginia Livingston and Gaston Naessens, who independently developed a similar microscope, saw similar events unfolding through the lens and, as a result, developed the latter's anti-cancer substance 714-X (see page 293).

Rife built a generator that emitted radiation of a particular frequency that destroyed the cancer-causing microbe. It was tested at the University of Southern California in the early 1930s. Rife reported the results: 'Sixteen cases were treated at the clinic for many types of malignancy. After three months, fourteen of these so-called hopeless cases were signed off as clinically cured.' The patients were treated every three days, which was found to be more effective than daily treatment, the reason being that the lymphatic system had to deal with the toxicity created by the dead particles of the BX virus. In fact, all the patients in the study eventually recovered. The machine had a one hundred per cent cure rate in cases of terminal cancer. If there is a cure for cancer this is it.

There is no doubt about the authenticity of the research – nor of the high quality of the scientists who participated in the study, who included a university president, a director of Northwestern Medical School, and other eminent doctors. The study was run under the auspices of the American Medical Association of Los Angeles, personally facilitated by the President, Dr Milbank Johnson. So what happened?

The story is that Morris Fishbein, a non-doctor who headed the American Medical Association (AMA), was also a front man for the pharmaceutical industry. Through his efforts, pressure was exerted on everyone involved to distance themselves from the machine. Some key supporters were bought off with large grants to allow them to retire in peace – and silence. At least two unnatural deaths occurred among key supporters of Rife – one was poisoned and another died when his laboratory burnt down. Equipment was stolen or tampered with. The manufacturers of the equipment were forced by various means into bankruptcy. Rife himself was taken to court. It was a mean and nasty war.

However, some doctors continued to use the machine. In 1940, Dr Arthur Yale reported the results he had obtained using Rife's generator. He reported on four cases that would have been fatal within ninety days. One was a fifty-three-year-old man with a grapefruit-sized tumour in the rectum. Within a week, the pain had gone and within sixty days the entire tumour had disappeared. Pain relief, it should be noted, is a possible sign that the cancerous stage of cachexia has ceased.

There appears to be no doubt that the machine worked. The underlying principle is that every living organism has an internal vibratory frequency – and that life without this frequency signature is impossible. If this frequency is altered, or if its power is amplified, then the organism can be destroyed. So the objective of the Rife generator is to

291

tune into the natural resonance of disease-causing microbes and then to increase the intensity of the frequency until they disintegrate.

Note that Rife used square-wave frequencies, not the normal smooth sine-wave form. Usually, the machine is used to send frequencies throughout the whole body – but it is also possible to direct the waves to specific parts of the body.

Proponents of the Rife frequency generator say that any illness from athlete's foot to yellow fever can be treated effectively using this machine. Usually, patients will sit for a period not exceeding forty minutes, with their hands holding metal cylinders and their bare feet resting on metal plates. The left hand and foot are hooked to the same output; similarly the right hand and foot. The patient then receives a sequence of specified frequencies, ranging from 1–10,000 Hz. The intensity of these frequencies is individually modulated, so that the patient will feel the pulse in the hand and wrist.

To begin with, in the case of an ill person, no more than four frequencies should be used in sequence. A healthy person, however, may be capable of experiencing twelve frequencies, one after the other, with no major side-effects. The duration for each frequency is from one to three minutes, depending on the level of health of the patient. Very ill patients must receive very short exposure to the frequencies, and should rest for three to seven days between treatments. For best results, the machine should not be used more often than every other day. This is because the toxic build-up from dead micro-organisms may grow too fast for the body to handle. Treatment is likely to last for six weeks to three months – and should be continued long after symptoms have disappeared.

A number of machines purporting to be Rife generators are on the market, but according to some critics, very few of them are worth buying. Some, for example, are machines converted from other uses. These tend to have poor quality components, and it is difficult to select precise frequencies and impossible to ensure that the machine emits the same frequency without drifting into other frequencies. Other machines suffer from the defect that they are pre-set by the manufacturer. This means you don't know what frequencies are being used and you have no control over them.

The features of a good frequency generator are that it allows personal tuning to a wide range of frequencies; that it has crystal-controlled tuning for accurate push-button frequency selection; that it has a memory so the sequences can be punched in and called up as desired; that it does not require the use of a transformer – transformers interfere with the high harmonic end of the frequency spectrum; that it can raise and sustain a 60-volt output; and that it has a pulsing device. It should have a UL544 listing – an American rating of safety for machines to be used connected to patients.

People undergoing Rife therapy must make sure they drink plenty of water before and after using the machine – and should expect to feel tired afterwards.

One helpful book on Rife generators is *Consumer's Guide to Rife Generators*, by Lyks Sieger and Dieter Reisdorf.[43]

714-X

This sounds like a new jet fighter, but is in fact a derivative of camphor, with an extra nitrogen molecule attached combined with organic salts. This substance was developed by French scientist Gaston Naessens, on the basis of his theory that cancer cells require high levels of nitrogen. In order to protect themselves from the immune system, the cancer cells release a substance which Naessens calls Co-cancerogenic K Factor, or CKF for short. 714-X neutralises this factor. This prevents the cancer cells from being able to hide from the immune system. The result is that the cancer tumour is gradually eliminated from the body by the body's own natural defence system.

714-X is administered by injection into the lymphatic system, usually in the groin area. A course of daily injections for twenty-one days is followed by a three-day rest before another twenty-one-day cycle. This continues for as long as necessary – for cancer patients, this usually means seven to twelve cycles. AIDS patients are also benefiting from this treatment. One patient, a Mr Ganong, on receiving this treatment, found that his tumour shrank so much after two months that his surgeon decided to operate. When he went in, he found the tumour 'had been changed into an apparently non-threatening jelly-like mass he'd never seen the likes of before', according to his son (quoted in Walters, 1993). Another patient diagnosed with metastatic prostate cancer in 1977 was cancer-free in 1989, after using 714-X. Some people suggest that the same benefits may be obtained simply by rubbing camphor-saturated preparations like tiger balm on the lymph nodes.

Information on doctors using this treatment and/or treatment with 714-X is available from organisations listed in Resources.[44]

Shark cartilage and liver
What is very impressive about the shark is that its immune system is very powerful. Wounds heal very quickly.

It is not quite the case that sharks don't get cancer – but it is almost true. Cancer is, it appears, very rare in sharks, skates, rays and other members of the elasmobranch family – which includes the dogfish. Why is this the case? According to Dr William Lane, who has almost single-handedly pushed shark cartilage as a cancer cure, the answer lies in the fact that sharks do not have bones. Instead, their skeleton is composed of cartilage, which has no blood vessels or nerves.

The cartilage contains a substance that inhibits the development of blood cells. Cancer tumours cannot grow without a network of blood vessels to nourish them. The development of a blood supply is known as angiogenesis. In normal adults, the blood network is already well developed. Angiogenesis therefore occurs in adults for specific purposes, ovulation and pregnancy, healing of wounds and fractures – and the development of cancer tumours. This would appear to indicate that wounds and fractures would take longer to heal if cartilage was applied to them. This is not in fact the case. It is well attested that cartilage speeds up the healing of wounds.

Bovine cartilage has the same effect, and was used in an experiment in the early 1970s. A concer researcher, Dr Prudden, administered bovine cartilage preparations to thirty-one terminal patients. In thirty-five per cent of the cases (eleven patients) a probable or possible cure resulted. A further twenty-six per cent had a complete response, followed by a relapse. These results were obtained with bovine cartilage, and shark cartilage is supposed to be a thousand times more effective as an angiogenesis inhibitor.

In addition to the cartilage, the shark's liver is believed to be full of other powerful, health-maintaining substances: it is a very rich source of vitamin A and it contains substances that promote healing and the production of white blood cells. It is therefore suggested that eating the whole fish – ground-up cartilage and all – could be a good way to a cancer cure.

The Chinese have been eating shark cartilage for centuries in the form of shark's fin soup. It is considered to be a rejuvenator and aphrodisiac. Shark cartilage is also supposed to be effective against arthritis, while helping to heal irritations and inflammations.

The problem is that shark cartilage capsules are expensive – and it appears that for cancer cure, long-term use would be required. As with herbs, they may keep things under control, but once stopped, the cancer may return. The alternative option, however, is to find a good source of fresh dogfish and eat the whole thing.

Unfortunately, Dr Lane believes that chewing and eating cartilage will not be very effective, as the digestive enzymes will break it up into its component amino acids and so lose the beneficial effect. To avoid this, shark cartilage can be absorbed through the skin via skin patches. Some believe that retention enemas, or taking the cartilage into the vaginal cavity, are more efficient ways of getting the compounds into the body – in that way they are absorbed without the presence of the digestive enzymes.

Each daily enema regime comprises two 15 gram doses in two-thirds of a cup of water at body temperature. In one study of eight terminal patients at a clinic in Mexico, using this protocol, the results were good. After two months, only one of the patients showed no response. The others showed tumour reduction of between thirty and one hundred per cent.

New research at America's prestigious Johns Hopkins University has shown that dogfish livers are rich in a hormone-like substance called squalamine, which has been shown to have very positive effects on solid tumours – especially brain tumours. This appears to be the active substance that inhibits the formation of new blood vessels. The liver is richer in the substance than the cartilage.

CONTRAINDICATIONS

Shark cartilage is contraindicated with the following groups of people: those who have recently suffered heart attacks, pregnant women, women seeking to conceive, people who have had major surgery, people on muscle-building programmes.

Sleep

Good sleep is important for health. Long-lived people tend to be good sleepers. We know that sleep is necessary for good mental health – dreams rest the brain. Sleep without dreams is not sleep, and sleeping pills inhibit dreaming. Sleep is also essential for good physical health. This is the time that human growth factor is secreted, and when damaged cells are repaired. The better the sleep, the better the repair.

For those who find it difficult to sleep, the following non-drug based approaches are recommended, either singly or together:

1. Add two to four drops of lavender essential oil to a warm, not hot, bath. Lie in the bath for twenty minutes.
2. Take 2–3 mg of melatonin before going to bed. If that has no effect, increase the dose by 2–3 mg, until you reach a level that has the desired effect. Melatonin is a hormone produced in the thyroid gland (see page 276). No toxicity problems are associated with it.
3. Take one or two capsules of the herb valerian.
4. Sleep on a magnetic bed (see page 226).

Spiritual healing

Many people have been credited with the ability to heal through spiritual or psychic means. This is often attributed to an ability to harness unconscious or telepathic forces. Often no explanation is to be found – certainly not a credible or proven one. But this does not mean it doesn't happen. Shamans use trances as a way of healing, and within their cultures they are highly regarded for their abilities.

Not all spiritual healing requires a spiritual healer. There have been a number of cases where people have recovered after having had some kind of vision. One remarkable, well-documented case was that of Dorothy Kerin, who at the age of twenty-three was a living skeleton, blind and waiting to die of TB, complicated by peritonitis and meningitis. One night, she had a vision in which an angel took her hand and said: 'Your sufferings are over. Get up and walk.' She had been bedridden for five years at this time, and her legs should normally have been too weak to support her. Nevertheless, she got out of bed and walked down the corridor. Her sight also returned, and in twelve hours her bones began to be covered with firm and healthy flesh. Kerin was so transformed by her experience that she became one of Britain's most famous faith healers by laying on of hands, until her death in 1963.

There is a network of spiritual healers in most European countries, including the UK and Ireland. It appears that some are highly receptive to human energies, and can read these radiating emanations in such a way as to discover and heal psychic, emotional and physical blockages. Some churches specialise in spiritual healings, and it may be that enquiries will lead you to a healer with a local reputation.

Spontaneous healing

Cancer tumours can disappear overnight, literally. When there is no obvious cause, this is known as spontaneous remission. It is universally accepted that this occurs, but there are differences of opinion about how often it does so. One standard opinion is that it occurs in one case in 100,000. Others believe it occurs much more frequently. One fifteen-year study conducted in California found 3,500 references to spontaneous remission of a wide number of illnesses in medical literature published in twenty languages. One of their conclusions was that spontaneous remission was widely documented, and therefore almost certainly more common than previously thought.

A Japanese study of spontaneous remission found a number of common features in the patients:

1. All suffered cancer as a result of an existential crisis.
2. On being told of their cancer, they displayed a complete lack of anxiety or depression.

3. They were all religious, and gave themselves up to the will of God – and got on with their lives in a sanguine frame of mind.
4. They all took measures to reconstruct their relationships with those around them.

There is even a patron saint for spontaneous remission of cancer. St Peregrine was a young priest who had a tumour in his leg, with the result that he was scheduled to have the leg amputated. The night before his operation, he prayed fervently. During the night, he had a dream that his prayers had been answered and that he had been cured. When he woke up, he saw that it was true. He went on to die of old age in 1345, and was canonised in 1726.

Some cases of spontaneous remission appear to be the result of intense experiences of emotional acceptance. In others, the tumour doesn't disappear – it remains, but does not grow. A state of apparent symbiosis results.

Sprouts

Not Brussels sprouts! Though they're good too. Here I refer to the freshly sprouted seeds of a number of plants such as adzuki, alfalfa, clover, fenugreek, lentil, mustard, radish, sunflower, watercress and others, including wheat, rye, millet and oat seeds.

Simple sprouting equipment can be set up at home to ensure a regular and extremely cheap supply of sprouts. These can be eaten as they are, or juiced with garlic.

The value of sprouts is that they are extremely rich in vitamins, minerals, enzymes and amino acids. In addition, according to advocates, they are 'biogenic', i.e. capable of transferring their life energy to the bodies of those who eat them.

Experiments with mice show that injections of sprout extracts have a strong inhibitory effect on cancer cells, and are completely non-toxic at even large doses. Lentil, mung and wheat sprouts were those tested with positive results.

Sunlight

Sunlight has been getting a bad press in recent years. Certainly, there is strong evidence to suggest that sunlight causes skin cancer (but only, some say, in those whose diet contains too much animal fat). But to conclude from this that the best thing to do is to stay indoors would be counterproductive. The fact is that there is also a very good correlation between high exposure to sunlight and low incidence of internal cancers. This beneficial effect is extremely important.

In one study, rabbits were exposed to different levels of natural light. The animals exposed to the most light developed the fewest tumours, had fewer metastases and fewer deaths. In a Russian study, animals exposed to sunlight had only half the number of malignant growths compared with controls not exposed to sunlight. A US Navy study, of cancer incidence amongst sailors, found that there was a relatively high incidence of skin cancer, but a less than average amount of all other cancers. The incidence of breast cancer in mice has been cut in half by exposing mice to ultraviolet light.

In one anecdotal case described by Dr Kime in his book, *Sunlight*, a forty-one-year-old patient had had a breast removed because of cancer, and had been given chemotherapy treatments because the cancer had moved into her lungs and bones. The doctors treating her were not hopeful of success. She approached Kime, who felt there was nothing he could do for her cancer, but that he could perhaps help improve her overall health. He removed the refined polyunsaturated oils and fats – particularly margarine, which is known to lower the immune system – from her diet and asked her to eat only whole foods, nothing refined. Dr Kime also told her about some of the research that had been done with sunlight and cancer. She acted on his advice and started to spend a great deal of time out of doors in the sunlight.

Before starting the sunbathing, she had been losing weight, but after several weeks of sunbathing and good dietary practice, her weight levelled off and she began to notice she had more energy. She eventually went back to see her doctors, and they could find no apparent symptoms of her formerly widespread cancer.

It is natural for us to visualise the warm rays of the sun as life-enhancing. We feel better out-of-doors in the sun. This is not an imaginary effect – the immune system responds positively to sunlight, and sunlight has been shown to increase the amount of oxygen in the body's tissues. High blood pressure is also correlated with high cancer incidence, and sunlight has the effect of lowering blood pressure – and so reduces the otherwise higher cancer incidence. So, all in all, a day pottering about on a beach or in a garden on a warm summer's day is a day well spent. And of course sunlight is relaxing and so makes the body better able to tolerate physical and mental stress. Sunlight, of course, is also very important for vitamin D intake. Foods supplemented with vitamin D are a poor substitute.

Some people are very sensitive to sunlight. They should instead increase their intake of carotene by drinking fresh carrot juice.

One of the ways in which sunlight is supposed to work is that it electrically charges the air as it passes through the atmosphere. Negatively charged ions are good for you and positively charged ions are bad. Heating and air-conditioning systems tend to increase the positive ions and take out the negative ions. The result is ill-health. Negatively charged ions increase your feelings of health, increased energy and mental and emotional exhilaration. Experiments with rats show that cancers grow faster if they breathe common indoor air as opposed to normal outdoor air.

Further evidence that sunlight is beneficial comes from a study that shows that New Yorkers who retire to Florida have lower cancer levels than New Yorkers who stay in New York.

Taking good care of yourself in times of trouble

It is known that physical and, more importantly, emotional trauma can lead to cancer. It therefore makes good sense, if you have experienced a traumatic event – the break-up of a marriage, the death of someone close or a business collapse, for example – to consider yourself at risk. At times like these, it pays to pamper your health needs. Book yourself into a health farm, have those colonics and aromatherapy massages you've always wanted but never plucked up the courage to do. Go to a naturopath and have a general health assessment done. Ease up in other areas. Allow yourself to be taken care of. Decide that you are important enough to pay this attention to yourself. Let's face it, you're worth it!

Urea

We've probably all laughed when we read of an Indian Prime Minister or a Chinese businessman extolling the virtues of drinking their own urine. But there are good reasons to suppose that it may be good medicine. Morarji Desai, once Prime Minister of India, lived to the age of ninety-nine, all the while extolling the virtues of a daily glass of his own urine. Chinese medicine and even orthodox Western medicine have similarly noted beneficial attributes to drinking urine.

One proponent of urine drinking is Hong Kong businessman Lee Hak-shing, who claims to have cured himself of a number of ailments including rheumatism, headaches, bladder stones and skin allergies. A Japanese doctor, Nakasue Ryoichi, explains this effect by noting that urine contains interferon, a natural immune substance found in the body – and which Western cancer researchers have been seeking, so far without much success, to demonstrate as an effective cancer-killing substance. However, some doctors, while not necessarily rejecting the urine thesis, feel that interferon may not be the active substance in urine – if there is indeed any active substance – because it would be digested by the stomach's gastric acid before it could be absorbed into the body.

At a 1996 conference on the benefits of auto-urine therapy (i.e. drinking your own urine), Dr Ming Chenliao of the Long Life Biomedical Company in Hefei province, China, made strong claims for urine's beneficial effects against cancer. He claimed that forty-seven per cent of cancer patients treated in this way were cured. At the same conference, Japanese researcher Dr Shigeyuri Arai, working at the Hayashibara Biochemical Laboratories in Okayama, Japan, claimed a success rate of seventy-three per cent with cancer patients. Over 200,000 Japanese gargle or drink urine every day, and this therapy is promoted by Japan's Miracle Cup of Life Institute. Urine therapy is reportedly also very popular in Germany.

While urine drinking may not be everyone's cup of tea, there appear to be very good reasons for thinking that urine is a possible source of health-stimulating chemicals. Dr Burzynski, who developed the antineoplaston therapy described on pages 232–3, derives his peptides not from blood but from urine. He says: 'Urine is not really waste material, but probably the most complex chemical mixture in the human body, and therefore it can deliver us virtually any information about the body. So from the cybernetic point of view it is just a treasure of information.' Blood is not such a complex mixture, as it contains fewer chemicals. So urine tests reveal more about the body than blood tests.

During the Second World War, British cancer researchers tested a urine-derived product which they called H11, and used it on 243 terminal cases. Forty per cent of the cases apparently recovered. However, what exactly this product contained is not known, as the research did not receive any support, and the details that have survived are very sketchy.

One of the major constituents of urine is urea. The average adult human excretes about 25 grams (1 oz) of urea a day. One Greek doctor, Evangelos Danapoulos, has treated cancers in and around the eye by injecting urea, with, he claims, almost complete success. Urea has no side-effects. In animal studies, urea has been injected directly into tumours, particularly melanomas, with the result that they regressed or were eliminated. While Danapoulos claims it is virtually non-toxic, American researchers suggest that the maximum concentration to be used should be forty per cent.

Urea can also be taken orally and this has, it is claimed, a strong beneficial effect on the liver and through that on the lungs. One way to distribute it more effectively to other tissues and organs is to mix the urea with creatine hydrate. This is the supposedly active ingredient of a much maligned anti-cancer drug known as Krebiozen. One test of the drug claimed that it stopped or reduced cancer growth in eighty-eight per cent of a group of 4,227 cancer patients, the vast majority of whom were terminal. Krebiozen was subsequently discredited, but still has its adherents.

To take urea orally, 15–30 grams of urea are dissolved in a quart of water. This quart is divided into seven portions. One portion is drunk every ninety minutes through the waking day. This can be taken with 3.5 grams of creatine hydrate, divided into seven portions of 0.5 grams, and eaten with a peanut butter sandwich or juice to mask its unpleasant taste.

Or you can, as many Indians, Chinese, Malays, Japanese

302

and others do, drink your own urine.

See Resources for sources of urea and creatine hydrate.[45]

Vibrational medicine

There is a thread linking many of the therapies already described – acupuncture, homeopathy, flower essence therapy, colour therapy, some bio-magnetic energy therapies, spiritual healing and prayer – with others not yet described: radionics and crystal therapy. For some writers, these are all expressions of a single, unified approach to healing, which can be called vibrational medicine, and which is based on principles opposed to those underlying mainstream medicine.

The key difference is that mainstream medicine deals with the here and now, with the physical body and its appearances, with physical, solid rules about physical causes and physical effects. This is a very Newtonian world. Vibrational medicine takes a very different tack.

For vibration medical practitioners, the body is not a simple, dense, solid mass of matter – on the contrary, it is an expression of energy. Their picture of the universe is that it is a single being – a unified energy system. Our bodies are ultimately nothing other than electrons and protons and neutrons whizzing about in space. They recognise, however, that there are different levels of being, and they distinguish various levels from the brute physical through the emotional and mental to the spiritual. There are a number of different schemes. The following is a standard example:

Mental Body (intelligence)
$\updownarrow$
Astral Body (emotions)
$\updownarrow$
Etheric Body (aura)
$\updownarrow$
Physical Body

Beyond the mental body there is a causal body, which itself is the progeny of higher spiritual energies. It is here that the casual reader tends to lose patience with the levels of abstraction, or become uncomfortable that a religious conversion is required. But if we restrict ourselves to the four earthly levels, we find something interesting.

According to this schema, disharmonies at higher levels express themselves at lower levels. All of these vibrational energy medicines seek to 'attack' these disease problems at levels higher than the physical plane. Bad thoughts do have bad physical effects. But since to 'cure' the body at the level of the body would leave the bad thoughts in place, it is necessary to deal with problems of disease at higher levels than the physical plane. Disease can also be prevented by paying constant attention to the higher planes. Bad thoughts and emotions are early harbingers of disease.

Each body is a body of energy. As such, it resonates at certain frequencies. These frequencies can be worked on at the energy level to promote health. Different beings, and different organs, resonate at different frequencies; so does the same being, in different states. Bach's flower essences, homeopathic remedies and colour-energised water are all filled with vibrations that work with these harmonious or disharmonious resonating frequencies. If two violins are placed at either end of a large room and the E string of one is plucked, the E string of the other will respond by resonating. This is because only those parts that resonate with the precise frequency will respond. The point, then, is to resonate ill parts of the body with healthy vibrations.

The acupuncture meridians and the chakra points of Indian medicine are points that link the physical with the etheric levels of energy. Stimulation of these helps the flow of energy between these two levels. Magnetism strengthens the aura, flower essences seek to resonate at the level of the emotions – just how total the emotions are can be remembered when we consider the difference in how we think and how we feel when we are blissfully happy and when we are depressed. The difference is total. In exactly the same way, the difference between illness and well-ness is total, as is the difference between nervous tension and total relaxation. The change from one state to another requires a transformation – which can occur spontaneously and instantaneously.

CRYSTAL HEALING

Crystal healers take as their starting point the belief that all matter is made of nothing but vibrating energies, which are aligned with the universal energies, and that crystals are forms that unify and focus these energies. During a crystal healing, any number and variety of crystals may be used and placed on the body – particularly on and around the chakra points, which lie on the central line of the head, body and pelvis.

A crystal healer bases all decisions about placement and arrangement of stones on his or her intuition. In fact, as with many other vibrational practices, the psychic sensitivity of the therapists is considered to be an important healing element in itself. Since the universe is a single energy field, it is argued, then each and every person is a locus for this universal energy. By aligning the healer's energies with the patient's, healing is aided.

Crystals are believed to have the ability to magnify energies. As well as being placed on chakra points and around the body, crystals can also be placed in water to create an energised gem elixir. This works along the same principles as the flower essence elixirs – though the latter are generally considered to be more wide-ranging in their effects. Crystals help to align mental and emotional energies.

Crystal healing devotee, Katrina Raphael, strongly recommends the crystal luvulite. She says: 'Luvulite is the pressure release valve that can bring peace and understanding to a mind and body that have lost their source of strength.' It helps the mind focus its own healing energies. 'This healing force, if properly used, has the power to heal any dis-ease and restore complete mental and physical health.' Unfortunately, luvulite is a fairly rare and expensive stone. However, all quartz stones have healing qualities

RADIONICS

Radionics is a more curious approach to healing. The practitioner uses a machine which has electrical and magnetic parts, but which is not plugged into any source of electricity. It is believed that this machine helps the therapist to align his or her psychic energies to discover the sites of disease by measuring the 'radiation' emitted from diseased tissue.

This system was developed by an American doctor, Albert Abrams. He noticed that various diseases produced a dull response to percussion. He theorised that molecules of diseased tissue have a different atomic and electronic composition from healthy tissue. Since electrons resonate, this difference at sub-atomic levels should be detectable. Subsequently, he argued that if the tissues could be made to resonate again at a healthy frequency, the disease would be forced to disappear. This is the basis of radionics.

As with colour therapy it is believed that therapeutic action can take place at a distance. There is, in fact, some support for such a theory in modern physics. According to this view, all reality has the qualities of a hologram; one prediction of this theory is that every part of the universe contains all the qualities and energies of the universe-as-a-whole – and is in constant flux with the universe. Changes to the universe will be manifested simultaneously with changes in the part – even if it has been removed from the whole. The reverse also is true – changes in the part will affect the whole. A hair, by this reasoning, retains its connection at the etheric level with the body's energy system, and can be used for both diagnosis and treatment. By treating the hair, the absent body is also being treated.

Apparently, radionics practitioners have been successful in this. Some healers use radionics machines for diagnosis, while using colour therapy for treatment.

Vibrational medicine is rich in possibilities. The therapies allied with it or based on its principles are largely free of danger. The promise of vibrational healing is that cures can be almost instantaneous. For further information, see *Vibrational Medicine* by Richard Gerber, and *Perfect Health* by Deepak Chopra.

VG-1000

This is an exciting new treatment invented by Russian immunologist Valentin Govallo. He discovered that cancer tumours have their own immune support system that switches off the immune system of the host body. So, instead of trying to strengthen the immune system of the patient, he looked for ways to attack the cancer's immune system.

Govallo found a substance, which he called VG-1000, in the human placenta that appears to act in this way. He has treated a number of patients in Russia. Of the first forty-five with advanced cancer, twenty-nine were still alive in 1996 – an extraordinary 64.4 per cent twenty-year survival rate. Expanded tests with 250 patients found that more than fifty per cent lived for more than ten years.

VG-1000 is not suitable for people with liver cancer, or whose cancer has metastasised to the bones.

People Against Cancer, an American activist organisation, are now conducting trials of VG-1000, in cooperation with the IAT Centre in the Bahamas (see The Burton approach).[46]

Virus against virus therapy

It is known that certain viruses have an anti-cancer effect – people have been cured of their cancers after natural infection with measles and also with viral fowl plague, sometimes known as Newcastle disease. In humans, the only known side-effect of Newcastle disease is 'pink eye'. A Hungarian-American doctor has studied this type of therapy with herpes and influenza viruses, producing exciting results. Influenza viruses have shown a strong protective effect against a cancer-like disease in experiments with chickens. Since Newcastle disease has the best effects, a live virus vaccine, called the MTH-68 vaccine, has been developed. Large clinical trials are underway in Hungary. Side-effects are not a concern. Most patients note subjective improvements in pain relief, but clear results have not yet been released.

The common mumps virus has also shown anti-cancer effects in Japanese research. It has been particularly helpful in reducing oedema (swelling of the lymphatic system – a common result of radiation), cancerous bleeding and pain. Tumour regression was also noted.

Visualisation and suggestion

The object of visualisation is to tell the mind what to think, and therefore to tell it what to do in the body. The idea is to let thoughts and messages filter from the conscious to the subconscious zones of the mind. Many athletes improve their performances through mental gymnastics. The mind becomes its thoughts – and so, too, does the body. By actively guiding the imagination, the body can be led to a state of health. If you want something enough, then simply imagine it over and over again while you are in a deeply relaxed frame of mind.

Some people may find this a difficult idea to accept. The story of psychiatrist Milton Erikson shows what can be achieved through thought alone. Erikson was paralysed by polio as a young boy, and forced to spend a lot of time on his front porch in a rocking chair watching the world go by. One day, left at home strapped to a chair, he found that he was too far from the window to look out. Suddenly, he became aware that his obsession with getting to the window was causing his chair to rock. He started to concentrate his thoughts on getting to the window. The more he did so, the more the rocking increased. He soon found that he could direct the movement of the chair by working on his thoughts. It took him all afternoon, but he managed to reach the window. This experience led him to the idea that he could influence other movements by concentrating his thoughts. Erikson was eventually able to overcome the paralysis completely and begin to walk again.

How can we use visualisation to help us stay healthy? By letting ourselves dwell inwardly on a healthy positive image. With eyes closed, for example, imagine your very favourite place. Maybe this is near where you live, or a place that you remember from your youth, or a place you have visited on holiday – it may even be a totally imaginary place. Wherever it is, it is a place where you are happy. Reflect on the happiness you feel being there. Feel the warmth of the sunlight. Feel the glow of the sun on your body. How comfortable you feel with the warm living rays of the sun permeating your whole body. It is filling your body with health and happiness, energy and love. It suffuses through all the limbs and through the whole of your being. With each breath, the warmth and the light grow stronger and lighter. You release yourself into the heart of this feeling, and sit and let your mind absorb these sensations. Then, when you're ready, you can return to normal consciousness.

This is just one example of the kind of creative visualisation that can, it is claimed, restore or maintain the body's health.

Some people visualise the cancer and watch as, in their minds, their body's immune defence system attacks and slowly destroys it. Some people focus their visualisation on the chemotherapy drug or the radiation they are receiving. They imagine the drug eating up the tumour. They imagine the radiation rays like the healing rays of the sun, dissolving the tumour.

Or, as one patient did, as golden bullets. This man had a form of throat cancer that was nearly always fatal, and it was at a late stage of development. He was given radiation treatment, but was not expected to benefit greatly from it – perhaps some short-lived comfort from a temporarily radiation-shrunk tumour. In addition to the radiation treatment, he was asked to visualise the radiation as millions of little bullets bombarding the cancer tumour. He also imagined the cancer cells as being weak and unable to repair themselves – while he imagined the normal cells as strong and repairing themselves quickly. He visualised the white blood cells swarming over the dead and dying cancer cells and carrying them out of the body through the liver and kidney. He did this three or four times a day. The result? He not only recovered, but suffered very little associated radiation damage.

The patient's doctor, Carl Simonton, had similar success with a large number of patients who were considered incurable. Of a group of 156 people, sixty-three were still alive four years later; in forty-three of these, the cancer had either disappeared, was regressing or had stabilised.

Some visualisation experiments have shown that volunteers can influence the numbers of various types of cell in the blood. A study conducted by Dr Jean Achterberg found that students who visualised having more neutrophils did indeed have higher counts of neutrophils by the end of the experiment, while those who focused on increasing the number of T-cells increased T-cell counts, but not neutrophils. This shows how powerful belief can be.

On the negative side, we can make ourselves ill by visualising the worst. Joan Borysenko calls this process 'awfulizing' – the tendency to imagine the worst possible consequence of any event. This tendency is often obsessive and habitual, a result of past conditioning: 'Awareness of our conditioning is the first step toward unlearning attitudes that have outlived their usefulness. Such awareness opens our ability to respond to what is happening now rather than reacting out of a conditioned history that may be archaic.' (Borysenko, 1987)

If we see visualisation as the right-brain imagination at work, suggestion is the intellectual-verbal partner. By letting them work together, we can harness powerful mental forces. Dr David Sobel, co-author of *The Healing Brain*, recalled how he was plagued by warts on his hand when he was young, warts that resisted all standard medical treatments. One day, his mother passed him an article from the newspaper. The headline was 'Warts Cured by Suggestion'. His curiosity aroused, he read on. In the article, he was told that hypnosis and suggestion could get rid of warts. He decided to try it out but, as they didn't explain in the article how to go about it, he had to invent his own method. 'I decided that I must concentrate intensely on the warts while repeating ten times (it had to be exactly ten times) the phrase: "Warts go away. Warts go away." I did this faithfully every day for about four weeks, at the end of which time [they] had all vanished.'

Dr Bruno Bloch, of Zurich, built a machine that had a noisy motor and flashing lights. He told patients to put their hands in the machine, until they were told the warts were dead. He would then add a pink vegetable dye to the wart and tell the patients not to wash or touch the wart until it was gone. Roughly thirty per cent of his patients were cured after one session. The relevance of this to cancer is this: warts are very similar to tumours. They are benign growths caused, like some cancers, by a viral infection. Anything that can work for warts has a good chance of working for cancer tumours.

Visualisation works. Cancer patients should make it work for them. The greater the visual, auditory and sensory involvement of all the senses they can bring to bear in the act of visualisation, the more likely success is to follow.

Resources

1. You can contact the National Headquarters at 2716 Ocean Park Blvd, Suite 1040, Santa Monica, CA 90405, USA. Tel: 1 310 314 2555; Fax: 1 310 314 7586.
2. Maggie's Centre is at The Stables, Western General Hospital, Crewe Road, Edinburgh EH4 2XU. Tel: 0131 537 3131; Fax: 0131 537 3130.
3. A service is offered by People Against Cancer, PO Box 10, Otho, Iowa 50569–0010, USA. Tel: 1 515 972 4444.
4. You can e-mail for free information on PDQ: cancernet@icicc.nci.nih.gov. Put the word HELP in the message heading, and ask for the information required. Or you can get in directly, through on-line services like CompuServe. You can also use the CancerFax system. Users dial 1 301 402 5874 using the handset on the fax machine. Then press the numbers on the dial following the voice prompts, to receive the information desired. Service is available twenty-four hours a day. Or telephone 1 800 422 6237 to speak to a counsellor who has access to PDQ information.
5. American Health produce an acidophilus powder which contains five acidophilus strains, including Lactobacillus bulgaricus. This is also available in liquid form. Enquire at health shops. American Health, Bohemia, New York 11716, USA.
6. SOD is available as Orgotein®, from DDI Pharmaceuticals of Mountain View, California. Also available as Lipsod®.
7. The placebo effect is very important and will be discussed elsewhere. Here, it should be noted that

mainstream medicine seeks as far as possible to eliminate it. This is partly because doctors see themselves as having two functions: as treaters of ill people; and as scientists helping in the broadening of knowledge. Doctors convince themselves that the second function is there to support and inform the first. This, however, can only be done at the expense of the placebo effect – which is a major gun in the armoury of all healers. Many doctors feel that it is somehow wrong to make use of the placebo effect – it is unscientific, therefore fraudulent. The patient, of course, doesn't care if the cancer has gone away as a result of a placebo effect. He is just damned pleased to be free of the disease.

8. Published by Slingshot Publications, BM Box 8314, London WC1N 3XX.

9. A multi-vitamin/mineral that has been developed by doctors at the Cancer Treatment Centers of America is called Immuno Max. Call 1 800 490 8555, or write to Shelby Health Systems, 3455 Salt Creek Lane, Arlington Heights, IL 60005, USA.

10. For particularly high quality vitamin C products, contact 1. Cantassium Ltd, 225 Putney Bridge Road, London SW15. Tel: 0181 874 1130. 2. Bronson Pharmaceuticals, 1945 Craig Road, PO Box 46903, St Louis, MO 63146–6903. Tel: 1 800 235 3200.

11. A recommended product is Original Silica, available from San Francisco Herb & Natural Food Co., 1010 46th Street, Emeryville, CA 94608, USA. Tel: 1 501 601 0700. Now Foods, 550 Mitchell Road, Glendale Heights, IL 60139, USA. Tel: 1 708 545 9098.

12. This can be obtained from Choice Metabolics, 1180 Walnut Ave., Chula Vista, CA 92100, USA. Tel: 1 800 227 4473.

13. Wobe Mugos Products, Enzymes and A-Mulsin (an emulsified form of vitamin A); available from: Mucos Pharma GmbH & Co., Alpenstrasse 29, 82538 Geretsried 1, Germany. Tel: 49 8171 5180. Pancrex V Forte, pancreatic enzymes, available from: Paines & Byrne Ltd., Bilton Road, Perivale, Greenford, Middlesex UB6 7HG, UK. Tel: 0181 997 1143. Good-quality vitamins (and miscellaneous items, e.g. laetrile) available from: Cantassium Ltd, 225 Putney Bridge Road,

London SW15. Tel: 0181 874 1130.

14. Send a large SAE to The Colonic International Association, 50A Morrish Road, London SW2 4EG, or telephone 0171 671 7136 for a list of registered colonic therapists in Britain.

15. For further information, contact The Gerson Institute, PO Box 430, Bonita, California 91908, USA. Tel: 1 619 585 7670. In addition, you can contact the Debra Shepherd Trust, Chapel Farm, Westhumble, Dorking, Surrey RH5 6AY. Tel: 01306 882865. This organisation provides information and support.

16. Kushi Institute, PO Box 7, Becket, MA 01223, USA.

17. Bristol Cancer Help Centre, Grove House, Cornwallis Grove, Clifton, Bristol BS8 4PG. Tel: 0117 9809500.

18. 1. Association of Green and Health, Daido Building, Room No. 303, 3-5-5, Uchikanda, Chiyoda-ku, Tokyo 101, Japan. 2. The Ann Wigmore Foundation, 196 Commonwealth Avenue, Boston, MA 02116, USA.

19. A pre-mixed high potency combination of flax oil, CoQ10, vitamin E and L-cytosine is available from Innovative Therapeutics, 2020 Franklin Street, PO Box 512, Carlyle, IL 62231–0512, USA.

20. Essiac may be obtained from Essiac Products Services, PO Box 1387, Fort Lauderdale, FL 33301, USA. Tel: 1 305 786 5221. See also the herbal suppliers below, 22.

21. Approach Gary Oden, Flat 2F, Vienna Mansion, 55 Paterson Street, Causeway Bay, Hong Kong. Tel: 852 2895 4247, for bloodroot ointment sources.

22. To find a herbalist in the UK, write to the National Institute of Medical Herbalists, 56 Longbrooke Street, Exeter, Devon EX1 6AH, or look up herbalists or health clinics in the *Yellow Pages*.
    For herbal suppliers, see the following.
    Neal's Yard Remedies, Neal's Yard, Covent Garden, London WC2H 9DP.
    East West Herbs, also at Neal's Yard, Covent Garden, London WC2H 9DP.
    GRAMS, Baldwin & Co., 171–173 Walworth Road, London SE17 1RW.
    Herbal Apothecary, 70a The High Street, Syston,

Leicestershire LE7 8GQ.
Phyto Products, 3 King's Mill Way, Hermitage Lane, Mansfield, Nottinghamshire NG18 5ER.

US Herb Suppliers

Brasseur's Herbs, 608 Hudson Avenue, Newark, OH 43055, USA.

Hanna's Herb Shop, 5684 Valmont Road, Boulder, CO 80301, USA.

San Francisco Herb and Natural Food Co., 1010 48th Street, Emeryville, CA 94608, USA.

23. Source of Lactobacillus bulgaricus (CH-3 filant): Christian Hansen Laboratories, Copenhagen 2100, Denmark.

24. Magnetico, No. 107, 5421 11th Street NE, Calgary, Alberta, Canada T2E 6M4. Fax: 1 403 7300885. Alpha-Energy Products, 7027 SW 87th Court, Miami, FL 33173, USA. Tel: 1 305 271 8815. Bluestone Clinic, London, UK. Tel: 0171 637 4533.

25. Immuno-Augmentative Therapy Centre, PO Box F-2689, Freeport, Grand Bahama. Tel: 1 809 352 7455. People Against Cancer, PO Box 10, Otho, IA 50569–0010, USA. Tel: 1 515 972 4444. For a fee, this latter organisation will send copies of your medical records to a large number of alternative doctors in the States and will then discuss with you over the phone which doctors have responded, the types of treatment being suggested and any other matter such as costs that may concern you. It is manned by volunteers.

26. Burzynski Clinic, 12000 Richmond Avenue, Suite 260, Houston, Texas 77082, USA. Tel: 1 713 597 0111; Fax: 1 713 597 1166.

27. Anyone with cancer wishing to request CanCell should phone 1 313 684 5529 Monday-Friday 11.00am-3.00pm Eastern Time. The phone line is busy and callers have to be persistent. Information about Can-Cell can be obtained from Nutrition Hotline, PO Box 840, Milford, MI 48381–0840, USA. Questions and correspondence should be directed to Vibrational Research Foundation, PO Box 265, Milford, MI 48381–0265.

28. Dr Keller, The Chronic Disease Control and Treatment Centre, Am Reuthlein 2, D-8675, Bad Steben,

Germany. Tel: 49 9288 5166. The drug can be obtained from the Carnivora Research Co., Lobensteinerstrasse 3, D-8646, Nordhalben, Germany. Tel: 49 9267 1662; Fax: 49 9267 1040. Other information on carnivora's uses against cancer, AIDS and other diseases can be got from: Morton Walker, 484 High Ridge Road, Stanford, CT 06905, USA. Tel: 1 203 322 1551.

29. Those interested in chelation therapy should contact: 1. Dr Shellander, 8 Chilston Road, Tunbridge Wells, Kent TN4 9LT. Tel: 01892 543536. 2. Arterial Disease Clinic, 57A Wimpole Street, London W1M 7DF. Tel: 0171 486 1095. 3. Send US $2 plus a stamped, self-addressed envelope to HealthSavers, PO Box 683, Herndon, Virginia, VA 22070, USA to receive an up-to-date list of chelating physicians.

30. Coley's toxins are available as a treatment at the following: 1. Dr Burton Waisbren, 2315 North Lake Drive, Room 815, Seton Tower, Milwaukee, Wisconsin 53211, USA. Tel: 1 414 272 1929. 2. Dr Klaus Kolmel, Universitats Haup Linik, von Sieboldstrasse 3, 3400 Göttingen, Germany. Tel: 49 551 396081; Fax: 49 551 396092. 3. Dr Guo Zheren, Paediatric Oncology, Beijing Children's Hospital, Nan Lishi Road, Beijing, China. Information is also available from Cancer Research Institute, 133 East 58th Street, New York 10022. Tel: 1 800 223 7874.

31. For referral to colour therapists, contact: 1. The International Association for Colour Therapy, 73 Elm Bank Gardens, Barnes, London SW13 ONX. 2. The Hygeia College of Colour Therapy, Theo Gimbel, Brook House, Avening, Tetbury, Gloucestershire GL8 8NS. Tel: 0145 383 2150. 3. Pauline Wills, 9 Wyndale Avenue, Kingsbury, London NW9 9PT. Tel: 0181 204 7672.

32. DMSO may be obtained from: American Marketing Inc., Rising Sun, IN 47040, USA. Tel: 1 800 367 6935. A doctor in Britain who uses DMSO is Dr Shellander, 8 Chilston Road, Tunbridge Wells, Kent TN4 9LT. Tel: 01892 543536.

33. Sound Healers' Association, PO Box 2240, Boulder, CO 80306, USA.

34. The British Homeopathic Association, 27a Devonshire Street, London W1N 1RJ. Tel: 0171 935 2163. The Royal London Homeopathic Hospital, Great Ormond Street, London WC1N 3HR. Tel: 0171 837 8833.

35. Hydrazine sulphate 30 mg and 60 mg tablets can be obtained without any restrictions from: Ms Donna Schuster, Great Lakes Metabolics, 1724 Hiawatha Court, NE, Rochester, MN 55904, USA. Tel: 1 507 288 2348; Fax: 1 507 285 4475. For further information, contact: Syracuse Cancer Research Institute, Presidential Plaza, 600 East Genesee Street, Syracuse, NY 13202, USA. Tel: 1 315 472 6616. Information is available on the Internet at: http://www.ngen.com/hs-cancer.

36. For further details about Iscador, write to: Hiscia Institute, Kirshweg 9, CH-4144 Arlesheim. The Hiscia Institute is attached to the Lukas Clinic.

37. Hufeland Klinik, Bismarckstrasse, Bad Mergentheim, Germany. Tel: 49 7931 8185.

38. Oral and injectible laetrile (B17) can be obtained from: Ms Donna Schuster, Great Lakes Metabolics, 1724 Hiawatha Court, NE, Rochester, MN 55904, USA. Tel: 1 507 288 2348; Fax: 1 507 285 4475.

39. Livingston Foundation Medical Center, 3232 Duke Street, San Diego, CA 92110, USA. Tel: 1 619 224 3515.

40. Chopra-style healing at The Practice, The Manor House, King's Norton, Leics LE7 9BA. Tel/fax: 01162 596 633. Maharishi Ayurveda Health Center, PO Box 282, Fairfield, IA 52556, USA. Tel: 1 515 472 8477; 1 800 248 9050.

41. Hospital Ernesto Contreras, 494 Calle Primera, Suite 904, San Ysidro, CA 92173, USA. Tel: 800 326 1850. Hospital Santa Monica, 4100 Bonita Road, Bonita, CA 91910, USA. The Bio-Medical Center, PO Box 727, 615 General Ferreira, Colonel Juarez, Tijuana, Mexico 22000. Tel: 011 52 6684 9011. The Gerson Institute, PO Box 430, Bonita, CA 91908, USA. American Biologics-Mexico, Admissions Office, 1180 Walnut Avenue, Chula Vista, CA 91911, USA. Tel: 800 227 4458. Addresses of other clinics can be obtained from: 1. Cancer Control Society, PO Box

4651, Modesto, CA 95352, USA. Tel: 1 209 529 4697. 2. Sally Wolper's survey *Tijuana Clinics, Where and How to Go.*

42. For information on uses of hydrogen peroxide for humans and for experimental agricultural purposes, send US $1 plus international postal receipt to ECH_2O_2 Inc., PO Box 126, Delano, MN 55328, USA. Ozone treatment: Biozon Ozon-Technik GmbH, An Der Haune No.10, Bad Hersfeld, D-6430, Germany. For information on doctors who offer intravenous hydrogen peroxide treatment, contact: International Bio-Oxidative Medicine Foundation, PO Box 610767, Dallas Fort Worth, Texas 75261, USA. Tel: 1 817 481 9772.

43. Further books are available from the World Research Foundation. Tel: 1 818 999 5483. For information on treatment: American Biologics-Mexico Hospital and Medical Center, 1180 Walnut Avenue, Chula Vista, CA 92011, USA. One brand of machine that claims to meet the exacting standards required is called the BioTech 2000. Contact Gary Oden, Flat 2F, Vienna Mansion, 55 Paterson Street, Causeway Bay, Hong Kong. Tel/Fax: 852 2895 4247.

44. Centre d'Orthobiologie, Somatidienne de l'Estrie (COSE), 5270 Fontaine, Rock Forest, Quebec J1N 3B6, Canada. Tel: 819 564 7883. Genesis West-Provida, PO Box 3460, Chula Vista, CA 91902–0004, USA. Tel: 1 619 424 9552.

45. Urea can be obtained from Bio-Tech, PO Box 1992, Fayetteville, AR 72702. However, they will only sell to doctors or health professionals but will ship to patients if a doctor so directs. Pharmaceutical-grade urea may be available through normal pharmaceutical companies. It is not expensive.

46. Full details of how to join the trial are available from People Against Cancer, Tel: 1 515 972 4444; Fax: 1 515 972 4415. VG-1000 is also available at the Max Gerson Memorial Center Hospital in Tijuana, Mexico.

Additional resources

Cancer organisations in the UK

Association of New Approaches to Cancer
c/o Park Attwood Clinic, Trimpley, Bewdley, Worcs DY12
1RE. Tel: 01299 861444. Can refer people to local holistic
self-help group and holistic practitioners.

BACUP
3 Bath Place, Rivington Street, London EC2A 3JR. Tel:
0171 696 9003. Info service: 0171 613 2121.

Centre for Complementary Health Studies
University of Exeter, Exeter, Devon EX4 4PU. Tel: 01392
433828. Can provide a UK-wide list of complementary
therapists.

Cancerlink
11–21 Northdown Street, London N1 9BN. Tel: 0171 833
2818; 0800 132905 (freephone helpline). 9 Castle Terrace,
Edinburgh EH1 2DP. Tel: 0131 228 5567 (admin). Offers
practical and emotional support and information for those
with cancer, their carers and families; also information on
self-help groups.

Council for Complementary and Alternative Medicine
Suite 1, 19a Cavendish Square, London W1M 9AD. Tel:
0171 409 1440. Can provide information on various aspects
of complementary medicine.

Marie Curie Cancer Care
28 Belgrave Square, London SW1X 8QG. Tel: 0171 235
3325.

International Federation of Practitioners of National Therapeutics
10 Copse Close, Sheet, Petersfield, Hants GU31 4DL. Tel: 01730 266790.

The following centres base their therapies primarily on nutrition and mind-body healing techniques. For people in financial need, there may be bursaries or arrangements with the DHSS that can make the treatments affordable. Enquire about this at each centre.

Bournemouth Centre for Complementary Medicine
26 Sea Road, Boscombe, Bournemouth, Dorset BH5 1DF. Tel: 01202 36354

Bristol Cancer Help Centre
Grove House, Cornwallis Grove, Clifton, Bristol BS8 4PG. Tel: 0117 9809500 (admin); 0117 9809505 (helpline).

Wessex Cancer Help Centre
8 South Street, Chichester, West Sussex PO19 1EH. Tel: 01243 778516. Also provides preventative advice for healthy people.

Park Attwood Clinic
Trimpley, Bewdley, Worcs DY12 1RE. Tel: 01299 861444. This clinic is run on Rudolph Steiner's anthroposophical approach. Iscador treatments are available here.

Natural Health Clinic
133 Gatley Road, Gatley, Cheadle, Cheshire. Tel: 0161 428 4980.

Cancer organisations in Australia and New Zealand

Australian Cancer Society
GPO Box 4708, Sydney 2001. Tel: 61 2 267 1944.

Anti-Cancer Council of Victoria
Keogh House, 1 Rathdowne Street, Carlton South, Victoria 3053. Tel: 61 3 9279 1111.

New South Wales Cancer Council
PO Box 572, King's Cross, NSW 2011. Tel: 61 2 334
1900.

Anti-Cancer Foundation of South Australia
PO Box 929, Unley, South Australia 5061. Tel: 61 8 291
4111.

Cancer Foundation of Western Australia
42 Ord Street, West Perth, Western Australia 6005. Tel: 61
9 321 6224 2365.

Victoria Chinese Cancer Group
North Yarra Community Health Fitzroy Centre, 75
Brunswick Street, Fitzroy, Victoria 3065. Postal address: 33
Winters Way, Doncaster, Victoria 3108.

Ian Gawler Foundation
PO Box 28, Darling South, Victoria 3145. Tel: 61 3 9572
3324.

Australian Natural Therapists Association
PO Box 308, Melrose Park, South Australia 5039. Tel: 61 8
297 9533.

Australian Traditional Medicine Society
PO Box 442, Suite 3, First Floor, 120 Blaxland Road,
Ryde, NSW 2112. Tel: 61 2 808 2825.

Cancer Society of New Zealand
PO Box 1724, Auckland, New Zealand. Information
service: Tel: 09 524 2628.

*Cancer organisations in Canada, South Africa
and Hong Kong*

Canadian Cancer Society
200, 10 Alcorn Avenue, Toronto, Ontario M4V 3B1,
Canada. Tel: 1 416 961 7223.

Cancer Research Association of South Africa
Cathe Kruger, Director of Corporate Communications, 26
Concorde Road, Bedfordview 2008, PO Box 2000, Johannesburg 2000, South Africa. Tel: 001 616 7662/9.

Hong Kong Cancerlink
Tel: 852 2323 2526.

Hong Kong Cansurvive (English)
24-hour hotline: 852 2328 2202.

Bibliography

Airola, Paavo, *Juice Fasting*, Health Plus Publishers, Oregon, USA, 1971

Anderson, R.A., *Wellness Medicine*, Keats Publishing, Connecticut, USA, 1987

Baker, Elizabeth, *The Unmedical Miracle – Oxygen*, Drelwood Communications, Indianola, USA, 1994

Barron, Philip, *Cancer: A Comprehensive Guide to Effective Treatment*, Element Books, UK, 1996

Benjamin, Harold, *The Wellness Community Guide to Fighting for Recovery from Cancer*, Putnam, New York

Bishop, Beata, *My Triumph Over Cancer*, Keats Publishing, USA, 1985

Black, Dean, *Health at the Crossroads*, Tapestry Press, Utah, USA, 1988

Boik, John, *Cancer and Natural Medicine*, Oregon Medical Press, USA, 1995

Borysenko, Joan, *Minding the Body, Mending the Mind*, Bantam Books, London, 1987

Brecher, Harold and Arline, *Forty Something Forever*, HealthSavers Press, Virginia, USA, 1992

British Medical Association, *Complementary Medicine: New Approaches to Good Practice*, Oxford University Press, UK, 1993

Buckman, Dr R., *What You Really Need to Know About Cancer*, Macmillan, London, 1995

Caprio, Frank S., *Better Health with Self-Hypnosis*, Parker Publishing Company, New York, 1985

Carter, James, MD, *Racketeering in Medicine*, Hampton Book Publishing Company Inc., USA, 1992

Chaitow, Leon, *An End to Cancer?*, Thorson's, UK, 1983

Chaitow, Leon, and Trenev, Natasha, *Probiotics*, Thorson's, UK, 1990

Chopra, Deepak, *Quantum Healing*, Bantam Books, New York, 1989

Chopra, Deepak, *Perfect Health*, Harmony Books, New York 1991

Cickoke, Anthony, *Enzymes and Enzyme Therapy*, Keats Publishing, Connecticut, USA, 1994

Clark, Hulda R., *The Cure for All Cancers*, ProMotion Publishing, California, USA, 1993

Compton Burnett, J., *The Curability of Tumors by Medicines*, Indian Books & Periodicals Syndicate, New Delhi (undated)

Cooper, Geoffrey, *The Cancer Book*, Jones and Bartlett Publishers, Boston, USA, 1993

Cousins, Norman, *An Anatomy of an Illness as Perceived by the Patient*, W. W. Norton & Co., New York, 1979

Culbert, Michael, *Medical Armageddon*, Vols. I–IV, C and C Communications, San Diego, California, USA, 1995

Davis, Patricia, *Aromatherapy: An A–Z*, The C.W. Daniel Co., UK, 1988

Davis, Ben, *Rapid Healing Foods*, Parker Publishing Company Inc., New York, 1980

Dawson, Donna, *Women's Cancers*, Judy Piatkus (Publishers) Ltd, London, 1990

Dermer, G., *The Immortal Cell*, Avery Publishing, USA, 1994

Desowitz, Robert S., *The Malaria Capers*, W. W. Norton & Co., New York, 1991

Dettman, Glen *et al*, *Vitamin C: Nature's Miraculous Healing Missile*, Frederick Todd, Melbourne, Australia, 1993

Dollinger, M. *et al*, *Everyone's Guide to Cancer Therapy*, Andrews and McMeel, USA, 1994

Donsbach, Kurt, *Oxygen*, Rockland Corporation, USA, 1994

Dossey, Larry, *Healing Words*, Harper, San Francisco, USA, 1993

Fere, Dr Maude Tresillian, *Does Diet Cure Cancer?*, Thorson's, UK, 1963

Feynman, Richard, *Surely You're Joking, Mr Feynman!*, W. W. Norton & Co. Inc., USA, 1985

Fink, John, *Third Opinion: An International Directory to Alternative Therapy Centers for the Treatment and Prevention of Cancer*, Avery Publishing, New York, 1991

Forbes, Alec, *The Famous Bristol Detox Diet for Cancer Patients*, Keats Publishing, USA, 1984

Frahm, Anne, *A Cancer Battle Plan*, Pinon Press, Colorado, USA, 1993

Friedberg, Errol, *Cancer Answers*, W. H. Freeman & Co., New York, 1992

Fulder, Stephen, *How To Survive Medical Treatment*, The C.W. Daniel Company Ltd, UK, 1994

Gerber, Richard, *Vibrational Medicine*, Bear & Company, Santa Fe, New Mexico, USA, 1988

Gerson, Max, *A Cancer Therapy*, Gerson Institute, California, USA, 1958

Goldman, J., *Healing Sounds – The Power of Harmonics*, Element Books, London, 1992

Goodare, Heather, ed., *Fighting Spirit*, Scarlet Press, London, 1996

Greenburg, Kurt, *Challenging Orthodoxy*, Keats Publishing, Connecticut, USA, 1991

Hagiwara, Yoshide, *Green Barley Essence: The Ideal 'Fast Food'*, Keats Publishing, Connecticut, USA, 1985

Harrison, Shirley, *New Approaches to Cancer*, Century Hutchinson, London, 1987

Hewitt, William, *Hypnosis*, Llewellyn Publications, St Paul, USA, 1994

Hirshberg, C., and Barasch, M., *Remarkable Recovery*, Headline, London, 1995

Israel, Lucien, *Conquering Cancer*, Penguin, UK, 1976, 1980

Jochems, Ruth, *Dr Moerman's Anti-cancer diet*, Avery Publishing Group, New York, 1990

Jones, Kenneth, *Pau d'Arco: Immune Power*, Healing Arts Press, Vermont, USA

Kaufmann, Klaus, *Silica: The Forgotten Nutrient*, Alive Books, Barnaby, BC, Canada, 1993

Kime, Zane R., *Sunlight*, World Health Publications, California, USA, 1980

King, Petrea, *Quest for Life*, Random House, Australia, 1992

Kushi, Michio, and Jack, Alex, *The Cancer-Prevention Diet*, Thorson's, UK, 1984

Lakhovsky, Georges, *The Secret of Life*, World Research Foundation, California, USA

Lane, I. W. and Comac, L., *Sharks Don't Get Cancer*, Avery Publishing, New York, 1992

324

Lang, S., and Patt, R., *You Don't Have to Suffer: A Complete Guide to Relieving Pain*, Oxford University Press, UK, 1994

Lerner, M., *Choices in Healing*, MIT Press, USA, 1994

LeShan, Lawrence, *You Can Fight for Your Life: Emotional Factors in the Treatment of Cancer*, Thorson's, UK, 1984

Liberman, Jacob, *Light: Medicine of the Future*, Bear & Company, Santa Fe, New Mexico, USA, 1991

Lieberman, S., and Bruning, N., *The Real Vitamin and Mineral Book*, Avery Publishing Group, New York, 1990

Lifton, Robert Jay, *The Nazi Doctors: Medical Killing and the Psychology of Genocide*, Basic Books Inc., New York, 1986

MacIvor, Virginia, and LaForest, Sandra, *Vibrations: Healing through Color Therapy, Homeopathy and Radionics*, Samuel Weiser Inc., York Beach, Maine, USA, 1979

McConnell, Carol and Malcolm, *The Mediterranean Diet*, The Bodley Head, London, 1987

McTaggart, L., *What the Doctors Don't Tell You*, Thorson's, UK, 1996

Mendelsohn, Robert, *Confessions of a Medical Heretic*, Contemporary Books, Chicago, USA, 1979

Mendelsohn, Crile *et al*, *Dissent in Medicine*, Contemporary Books, Chicago, USA, 1985

Milton, Richard, *Forbidden Science*, Fourth Estate, London, 1994

Mindell, E., *Earl Mindell's Herb Bible*, Simon & Schuster, New York, 1992

Morra, Marion, and Potts, Eva, *Choices: Realistic Alternatives in Cancer Treatment*, Avon Books, New York, 1980

Moss, Ralph, *The Cancer Syndrome (The Cancer Industry)*, Grove Press Inc., New York, 1982

Moss, Ralph, *Cancer Therapy: The Independent Consumer's Guide to Non-Toxic Treatment and Prevention*, Equinox Press, New York, 1992

Moss, Ralph, *Questioning Chemotherapy*, Equinox Press, New York, 1995

Mowrey, Daniel, *Next Generation Herbal Medicine*, Keats Publishing, USA, 1988

Passwater, Richard, *Digestive Enzymes*, Keats Publishing, USA, 1983

Pauling, Linus, *How to Live Longer and Feel Better*, Avon Books, New York, 1986

Pearson, D., and Shaw, S., *Life Extension: A Practical Scientific Approach*, Warner Books, New York, 1983

Pelton, Ross, and Overholser, Lee, *Alternatives in Cancer Therapy*, Simon & Schuster, New York, 1994

Raphael, Katrina, *Crystal Enlightenment*, Aurora Press, Santa Fe, New Mexico, USA, 1985

Robin, Eugene D., *Medical Care Can Be Dangerous to Your Health*, W. H. Freeman & Co., New York, 1984

Schechter, Steven, *Fighting Radiation and Chemical Pollutants with Foods, Herbs and Vitamins*, Vitality Ink, California, USA, 1990

Scheffer, Mechthild, *Bach Flower Therapy*, Thorson's, Rochester, Vermont, USA, 1986

Sears, Barry, *The Zone*, Regan Books, HarperCollins, USA, 1995

Shackleton, Basil, *The Grape Cure*, Thorson's, UK, 1969

Shelton, Herbert, *The Science and Fine Art of Fasting*, American Natural Hygiene Society, USA, 1934

Sieger, Lyks, and Reisdorf, Dieter, *Consumer's Guide to Rife Generators*, Uncommon Books, San Diego, USA

Simone, C., *Cancer and Nutrition*, Avery Publishing Group, USA, 1992

Simonton, Carl *et al*, *Getting Well Again*, Bantam Books, New York, 1978

Stein, Diane, *The Natural Remedy Book for Women*, The Crossing Press, California, USA, 1992

Thornton, Hazel, *The Challenge of Breast Cancer*, paper delivered at *The Lancet* Conference, April 21–22, 1994

Tisserand, Robert, *Aromatherapy*, Lotus Press, USA, 1988

Tisserand, Robert, *The Art of Aromatherapy*, The C.W. Daniel Co., UK, 1977, revised ed. 1994

Treben, Maria, *Health through God's Pharmacy*, Wilhelm Ennsthaler, Steyr, Austria, 1980

Tropp, Jack, *Cancer: A Healing Crisis*, Cancer Resource Center (self-published: 5880 San Vicente Blvd #103, Los Angeles, USA), 1980

Trull, Louise, *The CanCell Controversy*, Hampton Roads, USA, 1993

Vogel, H.C.A., *The Nature Doctor*, Keats Publishing, USA, 1991

Walker, Benjamin, *Encyclopaedia of Metaphysical Medicine*, Routledge & Kegan Paul, London, 1976

Walker, Martin, *Dirty Medicine*, Slingshot Publications, London, 1993

Walker, Norman, *Colon Health: The Key to a Vibrant Life*, Norwalk Press, Arizona, USA, 1979

Walters, Richard, *Options: The Alternative Cancer Therapy Book*, Avery Publishing, New York, 1993

Weil, Andrew, *Spontaneous Healing*, Alfred A. Knopf, New York, 1995

Whelan, Elizabeth, *Preventing Cancer*, Sphere Books, London, 1980

Wigmore, Ann, *The Sprouting Book*, Avery Publishing Group, New York, 1986

Willard, Terry, *Reishi Mushrooms*, Sylvan Press, Washington, USA, 1990

Questionnaire

This book has been written so that you can be prepared for a diagnosis of cancer. The questions below are to help you focus your thoughts about cancer.

1. How would you rate the likelihood that you will get cancer?
    A: 1 in 3
    B: 1 in 10
    C: 1 in 100
    D: 1 in 1000
    E: 1 in 10,000

2. What are your reasons for this assessment?

3. What could you do now that would improve your chances of not getting cancer?

4. Have you got any plans to implement the courses of action outlined in your answer to question 3? When? If not, why not?

5. If you were diagnosed with cancer tomorrow, what treatment or treatments would you decide to undergo or explore?

6. What strategy do you believe would be most likely to lead to your recovery?

Index

human papillomavirus (HPV) 3, 30
Humphrey, Hubert 79
Hunza people, Pakistan 184
Hutchinson, Curry 232
hydrazine sulphate 258–9
hydrogen peroxide therapy 279–80
hydrotherapy 260
hyperthermia (treatment) 88
hypnosis 123, 217, 260–61
Hypnosis (Hewitt) 261
hysterectomy 47, 92

iatrogenic disease 119–20
ICC (invasive cervical cancer) 46–7
ice-packs 102
Immortal Cell, The (Dermer) 110
immune system 30, 85–6, 102, 230–31
immuno-augmentative therapy 230–32
immunotherapy 35
Ingham, Eunice 288
intestinal cancer 22, 81–2, 190
intestinal fluke 29–30
invasive cervical cancer (ICC) 46–7
iodine 102–3, 167
iron 103, 150, 167
Ironside, Lady Audrey 75
Iscador 261–2
Ishitsuka, Dr Sagen 169
Israel, Dr Lucien 64
Issels, Dr Joseph, and therapy 262–3, 278

Jack, Alex 169, 171
Jenner, Sumi 218
John (cancer-prone personality) 206–8
Johns Hopkins Hospital, Baltimore 86, 110
Johnson, Mary 186–7

Jones, Dr Hardin 55–6, 63–4, 108
Joshi, Dr (Ayurvedic doctor) 203
Journal of the American College of Nutrition 172
Journal of Occupational Medicine 28
juice fasts 159–61, 177

Karposi's sarcoma 30, 93
Kaufmann, Klaus 149–50
Keller, Dr Helmut 234
Kerin, Dorothy 297
Keswick, Maggie 10
kidney cancer 93–4
Kime, Dr Zane R. 299
kinesiology 282
King, Dr Eileen 163
King, Petrea 217
Klopfer, Dr Bruno 211, 215–16
Kohler, Jean 171
Kuhnau, Dr (live cell therapist) 271
Kushi, Michio 169, 171–2

Lacks, Henrietta ('Helen Lane') 110
Lactobacillus acidophilus 103, 221–2
Lactobacillus bulgaricus 103, 221
laetrile (amygdalin) 263–7
Lakhovsky, Georges, and cure 243, 267–8
Lancet, The (periodical) 64
Lane, Dr William 2, 294–5
Lane, Helen (Henrietta Lacks) 110
Lang, Susan 25
language of cancer 34–5
lapachol (pau d'arco) 200–201
larynx, cancer 63, 149
laser treatments 88–9
laughter (treatment) 268–70

335